"*The Mindfulness and Acceptance Workbook for Anxiety* is so much more than the sum of its title. It's a way to live, a way of being, and a way of bringing kindness and compassion to our lives and to the lives of those around us. In short, this is one of the most beautiful guidebooks toward life—and living a more heart-centered, kind, and compassionate way—that I've ever seen. Take your time going through it, do the homework, and see yourself shine! We all have magic inside, just waiting beneath our worries and concerns. This workbook helps you move those aside—or technically befriend them, which is pretty amazing—to unlock the magic and help you shine brightly. Much more than a workbook, this is a kind and compassionate guide to life! I cannot recommend this book enough. It's a life-changer!"

—**Michael Sandler**, host of the *Inspire Nation Show*, and author of *Barefoot Running*

"You have in your hands a wise and healing workbook that is based on a radical premise: fighting or resisting anxiety adds fuel to the fire; learning how to relate to it with mindful presence and compassion leads to true well-being. Filled with accessible, well-researched exercises and practices, this guide can free you to live from your full aliveness, heart, and potential."

—**Tara Brach, PhD**, author of *Radical Acceptance* and *True Refuge*

"*The Mindfulness and Acceptance Workbook for Anxiety* combines the accumulated wisdom of the ages with up-to-date, cutting-edge developments in scientific psychology. In an easy-to-read and fun format, those suffering from anxiety in all of its guises will find the keys to breaking loose from its shackles. By emphasizing acceptance of toxic emotions (and illustrating ways to accomplish this) rather than struggling to overcome them, the person inside you may finally emerge to set your life on a new, productive, and valued course. Highly recommended for all those struggling with worry, anxiety, and fear."

—**David H. Barlow, PhD**, founder and director emeritus of the Center for Anxiety and Related Disorders, professor of psychology and psychiatry at Boston University, and author of *Anxiety and Its Disorders*

"This book presents a tried-and-true approach to turning your life in a new direction. If you want to stop running, hiding, struggling, or just waiting for your life to start, this book will help show you how to start living, now. Clear guidance, beautifully presented. Highly recommended."

—**Steven C. Hayes**, codeveloper of acceptance and commitment therapy (ACT), and author of *Get Out of Your Mind and Into Your Life*

"Ably surfing the dual currents of traditional exposure and acceptance-based treatments for anxiety, the authors of this resourceful workbook illustrate the synergies to be found in their combination. Carefully structured exercises and charts support the core message that taking action to face one's fears is most effective if acceptance informs our starting point, and values determine our destination. This book is a 'must-read' for anyone encountering anxiety as a barrier to leading a fuller life."

—**Zindel Segal, PhD**, distinguished professor of psychology in mood disorders at the University of Toronto, and coauthor of *The Mindful Way Workbook*

"Go into any large bookstore and you will find numerous self-help books, promising much. This one delivers. With a combination of sound theory, new research, deep professional involvement, clear values, and a joyful communicative style, this third edition of Forsyth and Eifert's highly acclaimed workbook is inspiring. Through principles of mindful self-reflection, acceptance, and compassion, the reader learns that the opposite of anxiety is not simply the absence of anxiety, but the experience of a more fulfilling life and a richer progression toward one's personal goals. At a time of much uncertainty, distress, and horror in today's world, this book offers a message to everyone—not simply those for whom fear is a specific barrier to personal happiness."

—**Ian M. Evans**, professor emeritus in the school of psychology at Massey University in New Zealand, and author of *How and Why Thoughts Change*

"If anxiety and fear is a major problem in your life, this book is for you. In this well-written and thoroughly researched workbook, John Forsyth and Georg Eifert will take you on a journey to regain your life. Using concrete exercises and examples, you will learn new skills to develop a different kind of relationship with your anxiety and fear. As a result, you will learn how to become more accepting and compassionate with yourself, and to eventually release the demons that have kept you from living a life worth living. Life is beautiful. Start this journey now."

—**Stefan G. Hofmann, PhD**, professor of psychology at Boston University, and author of *Emotion in Therapy*

"In this fully updated and expanded edition of their best-selling workbook, Forsyth and Eifert show how giving up your attempts to control anxiety and fear will help you to leave your anxiety problems behind and get on with your life. In the years since the first edition, a number of studies have demonstrated the benefits of the approach described in this practical and clearly written book. I recommend this new edition for anyone who struggles with anxiety."

—**Martin M. Antony, PhD, ABPP**, professor of psychology at Ryerson University in Canada, and coauthor of *The Shyness and Social Anxiety Workbook*

"Steeped in the rich tradition of psychological theory, *The Mindfulness and Acceptance Workbook for Anxiety* by Forsyth and Eifert represents a major advance for the practical treatment of anxiety and related conditions. This book will assist clinicians and patients in constructing a treatment plan that ensures progress in overcoming the many obstacles associated with conquering fears. A major contribution to clinical care, this workbook will contribute to the growing knowledge base on ACT, joining other evidence-based approaches as a major tool for treating the disabling symptoms that accompany anxiety. This reference book belongs in every clinician's library."

—**Terence M. Keane, PhD**, director of the behavioral science division of the National Center for PTSD, and professor of psychiatry and assistant dean for research at Boston University School of Medicine

"This is the definitive handbook for how to reduce the suffering that stems from anxiety-related problems. More importantly, the authors offer readers a perfect blend of lucidity, kindness, research-based knowledge, and concrete strategies such that readers walk away with the skills to live a successful life."

—**Todd B. Kashdan, PhD**, professor of psychology at George Mason University, and coauthor of *The Upside of Your Dark Side*

The
Mindfulness *&* Acceptance
Workbook for Anxiety

―――――― THIRD EDITION ――――――

A Guide to Breaking Free from Anxiety, Phobias *&*

Worry Using Acceptance *&* Commitment Therapy

JOHN P. FORSYTH, PhD
GEORG H. EIFERT, PhD

New Harbinger Publications, Inc.

Publisher's Note

NEW HARBINGER PUBLICATIONS is a registered trademark of New Harbinger Publications, Inc.

New Harbinger Publications is an employee-owned company.

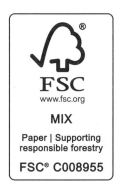

Copyright © 2025 by John P. Forsyth and Georg H. Eifert
New Harbinger Publications, Inc.
5720 Shattuck Avenue
Oakland, CA 94609
www.newharbinger.com

Cover design by Amy Shoup

Acquired by Ryan Buresh

Edited by Brady Kahn

Printed in the United States of America

27   26   25

10   9   8   7   6   5   4   3   2   1   First Printing

To our good friendship and support. With gratitude for thirty years of collaboration, fun, sharing, and learning from each other. Revising this book together was a pure joy!

—JPF and GHE

To my wife, Jamie, for her enduring love and support, and willingness to hold up the mirror so that I may see my blind spots and grow to become a better version of myself.

—JPF

To my mother, Margarete, who was a model of kindness and compassion to me through the way she treated everyone in our family. I know there were times when she didn't have the warmest or kindest thoughts and feelings toward us. But that never stopped her from treating us all with loving-kindness regardless of what she was thinking or feeling.

And to my wife, Diana: I am grateful and truly blessed that we can share our paths toward fulfillment with love, humor, and happiness—it is all within us.

—GHE

Contents

Acknowledgments

About sixteen years ago, we wrote the first edition of this workbook with a deep and abiding intention to help. At the time, we had no idea whether this workbook would be helpful and for whom. Now we know. We know because of the courageous efforts of readers like you. We also know because we tested the effectiveness of this workbook with people suffering with significant anxiety and depression.

We're grateful for the thousands of readers who took a chance on the first and second editions of this workbook, including those who offered us feedback and testimonials about the difference the workbook made in their lives. We also wish to convey a heartfelt thank-you to the 700 people, spanning twenty-five countries, who took part in our research studies to find out if this workbook works. You'll find a summary of what we learned in the prologue.

Writing this third edition wouldn't have been possible without the support of several people. We're immensely grateful to John's wife, Jamie, and Georg's wife, Diana, for their unwavering encouragement, sage advice, and loving support throughout the revision process. Their belief in the value of this book kept us going. We couldn't have done it without them.

The ideas and inspiration behind this book are not solely ours but belong to a broader community. This group of which we are proud to be a part is working diligently on the problem of human suffering and the promotion of well-being though an approach known as acceptance and commitment therapy (ACT, said as one word). This collective effort, fueled by research-backed practical skills, wisdom, generosity, and hard work, has deeply influenced us.

We are particularly grateful to Steven C. Hayes and the broader ACT community. Steve's journey with panic disorder and contributions, along with those of Kirk Strosahl and Kelly Wilson, laid the foundation for ACT and a pioneering book, *Acceptance and Commitment Therapy: An Experiential Approach to Behavior Change*, now in its second edition. Since then, ACT has mushroomed into a treatment with broad scope and solid research support. This new knowledge has guided us in writing this revised and expanded third edition.

We've also been touched and influenced by people beyond the ACT community. Pema Chödrön, Jon Kabat-Zinn, Jeffrey Brantley, Zindel Segal, Tara Brach, Sharon Salzberg, and others have echoed the core message of this book—meeting unpleasant emotions with patience, compassion, and acceptance. Their work teaches us that we can learn to let go of the ongoing struggle with anxiety and fear. This letting go creates space to show up to life and do what matters to us. This message embodies the ACT approach that we'll be sharing with you here.

We're also grateful to Kelly Wilson and our Swedish friends JoAnne Dahl and Tobias Lundgren, for sharing their work on values, such as the Life Compass that we adapted from their work (Dahl and Lundgren 2006). Thanks also to our British colleague Peter Thorne, who shared the "Anxiety News Radio" and "Just So Radio" metaphors with us. Joseph Ciarrochi, David Mercer, and Sara Christian contributed the wonderful hand-drawn sketches that you'll see throughout the book. We would like to thank each of them for kindly giving us permission to reproduce their work.

Special thanks also go out to the many professionals, students, and colleagues who have helped shape our thinking, and particularly David Barlow for his groundbreaking contributions to understanding the nature and treatment of anxiety disorders.

New Harbinger is a major outlet for the dissemination of newer third-generation behavior therapies such as ACT. We are grateful to Matthew McKay and all the New Harbinger staff for seeing the value of this work and its potential to alleviate a wide range of human suffering. We also owe a debt of gratitude and heartfelt appreciation to Catharine Meyers of New Harbinger for her tireless energy, encouragement, and kind support with this project, and to Madison Davis and Brady Kahn for their masterful, diligent editing and attention to detail.

Finally, we would like to thank the countless people who entrusted us to guide them on their healing journey. They, like you, were suffering with anxiety problems and finding it difficult to do what they care about in life. We've learned much from them, and their courageous spirit is present everywhere in this book. In so many ways, this book is a testament to their willingness to risk doing something new to get something new in their lives.

We've incorporated new exercises and insights in this third edition, aiming to empower readers like you to break free from anxiety and fear so that you can embrace and live your life to the fullest. This is our sincere wish for you.

—John P. Forsyth, PhD
University at Albany, SUNY
Albany, New York

—Georg H. Eifert, PhD
Chapman University
Orange, California

Prologue—Does This Workbook Really Work?

Research means that you don't know, but are willing to find out.

—Charles F. Kettering

There are many self-help books for anxiety problems. Most are written with good intentions. Authors want their books to be helpful. This was our intention too. But, honestly, we didn't really know. So we decided to do a research study to find out. As mental health professionals and behavioral scientists, we knew that doing a rigorously controlled research study was the only unbiased way to find out if our workbook is truly helpful.

By subjecting the book to scientific test, we knew there were only three possible outcomes. First, the data might show that our workbook is helpful. This, of course, is what any author would hope for. Hurray for us and you! Second, the data might show that readers are worse off after working with the book. This outcome would not be good for you or us. Third, the data might show that the workbook has no discernible impact; readers are no better off after finishing it than when they started. This latter outcome also would not be good. Despite the potential risks, we were willing to discover the truth, leading us to collaborate with others to test the workbook's effectiveness.

Here, we'd like to share what we learned and what it means for you.

WORKBOOK STUDY

The focus of this study was to see if the workbook makes a difference in the lives of people just like you (Ritzert et al. 2016).

We recruited an international sample of 503 people who reported struggling with severe anxiety and depression. Our research team then randomly assigned them, by flip of a coin, to either begin using the workbook right away for a period of twelve weeks or be on a waitlist for twelve weeks. After twelve weeks, we offered the workbook to those who were initially on the waitlist and monitored them for a period of twelve weeks too. We then followed everyone to see how they were doing six and nine months later.

You should also know that we had no contact with any readers in the study, so there was no coaching or therapist guidance. All we asked was that participants read and work with the material in the workbook on their own. That's it!

Improvements in Skills to Disarm Anxiety and Fear

As you'll find out, this workbook teaches various skills to help readers develop a healthier relationship with anxiety and fear. These skills include being less avoidant and less tangled up with difficult thoughts while learning to be present, flexible, compassionate, and accepting of internal experiences just as they are. In our study, we measured these facets of peace and genuine happiness at the beginning, after twelve weeks, and six and nine months later.

The good news is the results strongly support the benefits we mention throughout the workbook. Readers who used the workbook reported significant and meaningful improvements in mindfulness, self-compassion, and the ability to detach from unpleasant thoughts. They also became less avoidant and more accepting of anxiety, fear, and other unpleasant emotions. These changes coincided with using the workbook. Those on the waitlist showed these benefits once they started working with the workbook, but not before. Most importantly, readers maintained their improvements at the six- and nine-month check-in.

So, the bottom line here is one of justified hope. The results show that the workbook you have in your hands positively impacts the quality of people's lives by changing their relationship with anxiety and fear.

What About Anxiety and Fear?

As you read on, you'll see that we don't focus much on reducing anxiety and fear. There are two reasons for that. First, research and millennia of human wisdom teach us that there's no healthy way to completely reduce, eliminate, or avoid these feelings.

Second, science and human experience show that it's not the absence of anxiety that brings us more genuine happiness and peace. Rather, these qualities, including your freedom and sense of confidence, grow every time you do something that's important to you. That's why we focus on improving quality of life by helping you move toward your values. Still, we did look at what happened to anxiety and fear, and what we found is positive news for you.

Readers who worked with the workbook reported substantial reductions in anxiety, fear, worry, and depression. You may wonder how a book that doesn't focus on anxiety reduction ended up decreasing anxiety, fear, and worry as well as depression?

To get the answer, we reanalyzed the data using sophisticated statistical analysis (also known as multiple mediation). Below, we walk you through what we found.

What Accounts for the Good Outcomes?

Using mediation analyses, we discovered a crucial connection: the skills emphasized in the workbook directly contribute to reductions in anxiety and depression, as well as improvements in quality of life (Ritzert et al. 2020).

In fact, when you focus on learning the skills and cultivating a kinder and gentler relationship with your anxious mind and body, you'll feel better. It's the skills that lead to anxiety lessening, depression lifting, and quality-of-life improving. It doesn't work the other way around. Working to be less depressed and anxious doesn't lead to being less anxious and depressed, nor does it improve quality of life. Let this sink in, and linger with it a bit.

Reductions in anxiety and fear didn't happen by going after anxiety and fear directly. It was just the opposite. After learning the skills, readers experienced reductions in anxiety, fears, and depression, and ultimately improvements in their lives. This is an important message—one that supports the approach we offer in this workbook.

THE TAKE-HOME MESSAGE

We took a risk testing this workbook, and it paid off. Across the board, the results show that the workbook is helpful in many ways. But it only works for those who work with it. Readers in our study spent an average of four hours per week working with the exercises and material in the workbook, and most reported that it significantly changed their lives.

So, to benefit from this workbook you'll need to put some time into it. This investment will pay off, making you more adept at responding to anxiety and living your life. This is a point we stress throughout the workbook and another reason we return to old themes and concepts throughout. All the skills you learn must be nurtured and carried into your life from this point forward. They must become integrated into your daily life, not just tried and then forgotten.

To keep focused, we didn't spend time describing our second study, which compared this *Mindfulness and Acceptance Workbook* to a more traditional cognitive-behavioral workbook for anxiety (Russo et al. 2009). Nor did we cover another large study looking at the benefits of ACT for highly anxious people receiving more traditional face-to-face therapy (Arch et al. 2012). But these studies support everything we've shared with you here.

Many other researchers are also exploring ACT for anxiety and related concerns such as health anxiety, OCD, and PTSD. To date, the outcomes of this work have been positive (e.g., Bluett et al. 2014; Caletti et al. 2022; Coto-Lesmes, Fernández-Rodríguez, and González-Fernández 2020; Hoffmann et al. 2021; Ivanova et al. 2016; Philip and Cherian 2021; Ruiz et al. 2020; Swain et al. 2013; Twohig and Levin 2017; Wharton et al. 2019).

We know there's more work to do, but you can be confident in knowing that you're not walking into uncharted territory. Evidence supporting ACT for anxiety and many other human concerns is strong and growing. You too can find genuine happiness and get your life moving in ways that matter to you. Now it's time to commit to doing that important work yourself.

Introduction

There are two primary choices in life:
to accept conditions as they exist,
or accept the responsibility for changing them.

—Denis Waitley

We'd like to start off with a simple yes-or-no question. Read it slowly, but don't read into it. Listen to your gut. This isn't about labeling yourself with a diagnosis. We're not asking you to judge yourself either. Just answer honestly yes or no. That's it. Now, here's the question:

Is anxiety and fear a major problem in your life?

If you answered yes, you're not alone. If you answered no, you're in good company too. But if you answered yes, then you're probably suffering in some way. It's not that you just have anxiety. You have a problem with anxiety.

You may be suffering from anxiety, fears, panic, unsettling thoughts, painful memories, and worry. More deeply, you may know that anxiety has hurt you and your life. You may feel frustrated, exhausted, broken, damaged, and at your wit's end. You're looking for a way out. You may even think something is wrong with you. Again, you're not alone.

FREEDOM FROM ANXIETY MANAGEMENT

There's no way to escape the simple fact that anxiety is part of life. The emphasis here is on the word "part." You may feel differently. For you, anxiety may feel like it has taken over and become your life. But it doesn't have to be this way.

For many, anxiety is not a problem but an unpleasant and inevitable part of being human. You may wonder how people manage to do this, even when they experience significant anxiety and fear. Here's what they do. They don't put all their time, attention, energy, and resources into trying to cope with, manage, or resist thinking and feeling anxious or afraid. Instead, they put their energy into doing what matters most to them—with or without anxiety and fear. In short, they've learned not to let anxiety and fear dictate what they do. You can get there too.

This simple idea points the way out of anxiety and back into your life. Anxiety need not continue to cause you to suffer by putting a choke hold on you and your life. There's another way: a set of skills that we'll help you learn, so you can devote more of your energies to aspects of your life that matter to you. This book, supported by solid research, will help you get to a place where anxiety and fear no longer control you.

If you're like most people, then you know how difficult it is to get a handle on anxiety. And you've probably done many different things already to manage or reduce your panic, fears, worries, and tension. The activity below will help you get a better sense of this.

Here, you'll find a list of some common things people do when they struggle with anxiety and fear. Look it over. Place a check mark (✔) in the box next to the strategies that you've tried.

☐ Running away from situations that make me feel scared, anxious, or nervous

☐ Avoiding activities or situations that may trigger anxious thoughts, feelings, and memories (e.g., going outside, driving, working, being in a crowd, being alone, experiencing a new situation, eating certain foods, exercising)

☐ Suppressing or pushing out disturbing thoughts and feelings

☐ Distracting myself from anxiety, fear, and worrisome thoughts

☐ Changing how I think—replacing the "bad" thoughts with "good" thoughts

☐ Talking myself out of anxiety, panic, fear, or worry

☐ Sticking close to "safe" people (e.g., friend, family member)

☐ Overeating or undereating to soothe myself

☐ Sleeping too much or avoiding sleep so as to avoid feeling anxious

☐ Carrying objects or performing rituals (e.g., phoning, checking, counting, cleaning, washing)

☐ Talking or venting with a friend or family member about my anxiety

☐ Joining online support groups for people with anxiety problems

☐ Educating myself by reading books written by experts on anxiety disorders

☐   Turning to self-help books offering "better" ways to control worry, anxiety, and fear

☐   Using antianxiety medications, herbal supplements, or other recreational drugs (e.g., marijuana, alcohol) to dull the pain

Don't fault yourself for checking one or more boxes. Many people do. The strategies seem reasonable. They also tend to be followed by short-term relief. So, if you panic in the mall and run out to the parking lot, you'll likely feel better once you're outside. This is the great seduction of avoidance. You get a brief hiatus from anxiety and fear.

But wait a minute. Aren't you looking for a lasting, long-term solution? Does fleeing a panic-inducing situation make the panic go away for good? If it did, we'd probably tell you to keep doing it. But that's not how it works. Avoidance, escape, coping, and the countless other strategies people try do not work. In fact, leaving situations when you feel panicky or anxious often comes with its own set of costs. With the mall example, one cost might include not buying that gift you were looking for. Shame, guilt, embarrassment may be part of it too. Costs such as these are often associated with the very strategies people use to deal with their anxieties and fears.

To see for yourself, look at the boxes you checked from the list above. Have any of these strategies worked for you in the long run? Or have they cost you in some way? For now, see if you can connect with at least one of the costs in your life. Have you missed out on anything because you've been busy trying to avoid feeling anxious or afraid? Think about something you really care about, however small or big. Perhaps it's work, finances, or family. Maybe it's travel, exercise, a hobby, or your health. Or it may involve relationships, intimacy, your freedom, peace of mind, or spirituality. Take a moment and write that one important thing below. We'll come back to this later.

I have missed out on or am unable to _____

_____ because of my anxious thoughts and feelings.

Anxiety and fear are intense and action-oriented emotions that are hard to control in any permanent sense. Your lived experiences up to this point probably tell you as much. The truth is that anxiety may never go away entirely. As much as we'd like to tell you otherwise, there's no magical solution that will remove anxiety and fear from your life. Why?

Because we're historical creatures. Modern neuroscience teaches us as much. Our nervous systems are additive, not subtractive. This means that what goes in, stays in, short of brain insult or injury. Right now, you probably have a history that creates a good deal of anxiety and fear. Part of your history also has taught you how to deal with it. It's all in the mix. The good news is that you can change the mix and get your life back. We'll teach you how.

OVERVIEW OF THE JOURNEY AHEAD

This book will take you on a journey that will challenge you in many ways. As your guides, we know what lies ahead, and we have taken many people just like you on this new adventure. We also understand that the journey may seem a bit strange, even scary at times. But if you stick with it and trust us—and do the work—your life will change for the better.

Inside the "anxiety is a problem" mindset is often a relationship with anxiety that's hostile and unkind. This simply feeds and strengthens anxiety. And, as anxiety grows, you'll tend to struggle with it and resist it more—and on and on it goes in an endless cycle.

This is why we're going to show you ways to change your relationship with anxiety, yourself, and the history you've had up to this point. This includes how you respond to thoughts, memories, and images that trigger anxiety, the uncomfortable and scary feelings themselves, and your natural inclination to try to make it stop or to avoid it all together.

As you'll learn, developing acceptance and compassion for the more painful parts of your inner emotional life will weaken the power of anxiety to keep you stuck and suffering. This will allow you to create space to discover, or perhaps rediscover, what you want to be about in this life and where you want to go. As that space grows, you'll refocus your energies on the people and experiences that matter most to you. You'll find that the things you spend your time doing will change. New possibilities will emerge. In those moments, you no longer have a problem with anxiety. You're living your life.

Nobody wants to be about anxiety now and forevermore. Yet this is what you can become, so long as anxiety is met with negative energy. That negative energy is packaged in the form of active resistance, denial, struggle, suppression, avoidance, and escape. As you read this book and do the exercises, you'll learn why this is so.

These ideas are not fluff. They're backed by a growing research base showing that anxiety management and control feeds anxiety and fear, shrinks lives, and promotes suffering that you know about firsthand (e.g., Conroy et al. 2020; De Castella et al. 2018; Dryman and Heimberg 2018; Eifert and Heffner 2003; Eifert, McKay, and Forsyth 2006; Hayes 2004; Hayes, Follette, and Linehan 2004; Hayes et al. 2006; Hayes, Strosahl, and Wilson 2016; Salters-Pedneault, Tull, and Roemer 2004; Strauss, Kivity, and Huppert 2019; Yadavaia, Hayes, and Vilardaga 2014).

This is why we're not going to teach you new ways to control or regulate your anxiety. Instead, we'll help you learn to control what you can control. This will increase your vitality and ability to create a full life, free of the pain of ongoing struggle with anxiety. As you do more of that, you can expect to think and feel better too. Curious? Suspicious? Good—read on.

HOW TO USE THIS BOOK

The exercises are the most important part of this book. You need to do something with the material. We can't stress this enough. Doing the exercises will teach you new skills. Repetition will turn these skills into habits, changing your life trajectory. Reading this book, without doing anything with the material, may lead to new insights and wisdom, but that alone isn't enough. True transformation comes from your active participation. To make the most of this book, you need to work with it. Here's how:

- **Put taking care of yourself on your to-do list.** Set an intention to use this workbook. Consider whether you and your life are as important as the mundane tasks on your to-do list each day. We think you're important enough to be at the top of such a list. So put taking care of yourself on your to-do list every day.

- **Make reading a priority.** Commit to it! Set aside a reasonable amount of time each week to read this book. Be flexible. If you planned on reading in the morning and missed that reading time for whatever reason, allow yourself time to do it later.

- **Practice the exercises.** This is how you'll learn new skills, so you can respond to your anxieties, fears, and your life in new ways. Learning any new skill takes time. Every time you practice one of the exercises, you'll weaken old habits that have kept you stuck and miserable. You just need to do the exercises and see which ones work best for you.

- **Be patient with yourself.** Change takes time. We understand the urgency to fix things quickly, but getting a different outcome in your life can't be done overnight. We strongly recommend resisting the temptation to read several chapters at once, because you may end up feeling overwhelmed and it will be hard to practice applying the new concepts and skills in your life. You need time to think about and work with the material—let it seep in. Be patient with yourself.

- **Pace yourself.** To get the most out of this book, aim to read one chapter per week and practice the exercises daily or every other day. The chapters in part 1 can be read more quickly, but when you get into parts 2 and 3, slow things down! We've structured the book to be read this way. Take as much time as you need with the material in each chapter. Don't move on too quickly; instead, trust your experience. When you feel confident applying the new skills in your life, you're ready to move on. Let your progress guide your pace.

- **Concepts and themes are repeated for a reason.** Repetition is your clue that a concept or skill is important. The point is not to read and forget, even though many people do just that with self-improvement books. We miss how skills apply to new challenges unless we're taught to make the connection. Our intention is not just to inspire you but to change you for the better. If we could be with you in person as you use this workbook, then we would also regularly return to earlier themes and concepts. Why? Because you'll likely slip into old unhelpful habits and behavior patterns over time. That's perfectly normal. So, embrace repetition—think, "familiar-sounding themes are important themes." The challenge is to make them a habit in your life. That takes repetition, commitment, and practice.

- **Use the resources available for this book.** Worksheets for some of the exercises are included in the workbook and can also be downloaded freely by visiting New Harbinger's workbook companion website at http://www.newharbinger.com/54476. Use the website to print out as many clean copies of a worksheet as needed for your personal use. We also highly recommend downloading and listening to the audio versions of some key exercises. Online worksheets and audio resources are clearly marked with the icon shown here:

- **Use the workbook on your own or as a part of therapy.** This book was written to help anyone who may be struggling with anxiety problems, in whatever forms they may take. You don't need to have an anxiety disorder to benefit from this workbook. You don't need to be working with a therapist, either. Still, we've found that this workbook can be helpful when used along with therapy, but do check in with your therapist first. Therapists with experience and training in newer cognitive behavioral therapies, such as acceptance and commitment therapy (ACT), will know the content of this workbook inside and out. If you're currently seeing an ACT therapist, you may find that the chapters roughly correspond to what you're doing in therapy. If you're looking for an ACT therapist, you can find one at http://www.contextualscience.org/act_for_the_public.

OUR JOURNEY: WHY WE WROTE THIS BOOK

This book contains the best of what we know is helpful for anxiety and related problems. Many paths led us to write this book. Here, we'd like to share a bit about us and our journey.

As clinical psychologists and researchers, we've specialized in traditional cognitive behavioral therapy (tCBT). We've also dedicated ourselves to unraveling the roots of anxiety and anxiety disorders and how they can be effectively treated. More broadly, we're passionate about finding better ways to enhance psychological well-being and alleviate human suffering.

It's common for people with anxiety concerns to get better—meaning less anxious—with tCBT, only to return to therapy for more help later on. We've seen that pattern too. Often, people come back after successful therapy because their anxiety and fears have returned. This partial or full recurrence of anxiety after tCBT is more common than many would like to believe.

Many people seeking relief from anxiety problems have been through the mill of sensible strategies, often with limited success. Something there didn't seem right to us. And, as we stepped back, we began to question whether tCBT was promoting an unhelpful message. That message is this: anxious thoughts and feelings are the problem and keep you from creating a better, richer, and more meaningful life. If that's so, then the only way you'll have a better life is if you first take care of your anxiety. Often this involves learning ways to control and change what you think, feel, and remember.

This approach also suggests that it's not okay to be you. Or, put another way, it's not okay to have the history you've already had up to this point in your life. And along with that comes the idea that it's not okay to think what you think and feel what you feel. Many people seeking therapy initially share this belief, at least early on. Many therapies for anxiety problems promote this message by focusing on changing thoughts and feelings—and when and if you're successful doing that, you'll be happy and thrive.

But the message that it's not okay to be you still lives inside this approach. And that message itself is hurtful. There's just no healthy way to go forward while holding on to the idea that something is fundamentally wrong with you and your genuine emotional experiences.

Over the years, both of us have learned a thing or two about anxiety and how to treat it. But we haven't escaped the darker side of anxiety and fear. In truth, both of us have gotten stuck trying to get a handle on our mental and emotional pain. Early on, we turned to our trusted bag of tCBT strategies. However, they didn't seem to work well in the long run. So even the two of us—the anxiety experts—couldn't get rid of our anxiety. And you know something? That's okay. Getting anxiety under control is no guarantee of a meaningful life or genuine happiness.

By the early 1990s, a groundbreaking approach emerged, one offering a counterintuitive alternative to tCBT's focus on anxiety management and control. In fact, it went so far as to claim that control is not the solution for anxiety but the problem. This radical idea spurred a wave of research that included many scientists and therapists, culminating in the birth of ACT. Inspired by this new approach, we reevaluated how we address anxiety-related concerns.

As the evidence mounted, both of us pivoted away from promoting anxiety management and control. Instead, we began teaching people how to let go of trying to control, fix, or manage anxiety. We taught people how to be open to their genuine emotional experiences. The idea wasn't to get people to be open to their thoughts, memories, and emotions, just for the sake of it. Teaching people to let go of their needless struggle with anxiety created an opening. In that opening, we focused on helping people exercise control where they have it.

As you'll learn, we can control how we respond to whatever our minds, bodies, and emotions offer us, and we can control what we do to support the person we wish to be and the kind of life we wish to live. This very simple idea blossomed into a powerful set of research-supported strategies and skills to help people bring acceptance, compassion, and gentleness to their unpleasant thoughts, feelings, memories, and even their sense of self. Struggling to think and feel better was no longer part of the anxiety solution. The solution now focused on helping people change their relationship with their emotional life while also learning how to live well with whatever they might be feeling or thinking. A radical idea? You bet!

ACT is part of this new approach and forms the fabric of the ideas we'll be sharing with you in this book. We've spent a good part of our careers expanding ACT to help people just like you. We've also been using it in our daily lives—at work, with our kids, in our relationships, with our health, in our communities, and while doing things we enjoy.

We're not saying any of this is easy. It takes practice and commitment. But the payoff can be profoundly life altering. Our lives have been enriched in so many ways simply because we've learned how to put our energies to good use. We're less caught up in our suffering minds and more engaged in doing what we care about. And we've seen this work with those who have sought our help, including thousands of people who have used this book.

Our intention is to help you make the most of your one precious life. This workbook is here to help you on your way. If you give it a real chance, we think you'll be pleasantly surprised. Your life will be better for it too.

BEGIN YOUR JOURNEY

This book is designed to help you get something different by doing something different. Reading this book—and internalizing what you learn—is part of this process. But there's no book on the planet, no pill or person, that can make you live your life in a certain way. It'll be up to you to put what you learn into action to make the changes you need to make. In the end, you control the direction you want your life to take—that's your choice.

You've probably heard the Buddhist saying that the journey of a thousand miles begins with a single step. Getting your hands on this book is a step in a new direction. Reading this book, even up to this point, is yet another step on your journey out of anxiety and into a new life. Congratulations on getting this far!

The harder part is taking consistent steps to keep yourself moving forward.

A life lived well is the product of many small moments, not all of them pleasant. It takes a lifetime to create a life. Living according to your values is something we'll help you do more of, one step at a time. On your journey, you'll learn, progress, and see life in a way that you may never have experienced before. The important thing is that you are taking steps, for even baby steps will eventually take you up a mountain.

We invite you to make this book your travel guide. Use the information here to help you decide where you want to go. As you commit to putting your values into action, the quality of your life, and of those around you, will begin to improve.

PART 1

Preparing the Way for Something New

Your life is a sacred journey. And it is about change, growth, discovery, movement, transformation, continuously expanding your vision of what is possible, stretching your soul, learning to see clearly and deeply, listening to your intuition, taking courageous challenges at every step along the way. You are on the path exactly where you are meant to be right now. And from here, you can only go forward, shaping your life story into a magnificent tale of triumph, of healing, of courage, of beauty, of wisdom, of power, of dignity, and of love.

—Caroline Joy Adams

CHAPTER 1

Choose a New Approach

In any given moment we have two options:
to step forward into growth or step back into safety.

—Abraham Maslow

This chapter is about preparing the way for something new in your life. We recognize that we're all creatures of habit. Often, we repeat the same behaviors and patterns of thinking even though they're unhelpful.

We may even try harder while hoping that somehow things will change for the better. Of course, there's something to be said for hard work and persistence, but that's not what we're talking about here. We're also not talking about experimenting—learning from the past and tweaking what you do going forward.

What we're talking about is the tendency to get into a rut of doing the same old thing expecting a different outcome. We do not want to do that here.

To get a different outcome, you need to change what you're doing *now*. We've put this simple idea in the form of a mantra to help you remember:

If I continue to do what I've always done, then I'm going to get what I've always got.

If I am willing to do something new, then I might get something new.

Write it down and keep it with you as you work with the material in this book.

YOU HAVE CHOICES

You have the power to make choices. In fact, most moments in life involve making some kind of choice or decision. But having anxiety isn't one of them. Anxiety happens. It's not a choice. Nobody chooses to be anxious or afraid. But you can decide how you respond.

As Abraham Maslow teaches us, you can choose "to step back into safety" when anxiety shows up. Or, you can choose to do something new, which may help you grow and alter the trajectory of your life in ways that may have seemed impossible until now.

The material in this book will teach you how to respond differently to anxiety and your life by putting you in control of what you can control. Here are some examples highlighting what this book will help you do. Each example also involves a choice:

- You can choose to stop putting all your attention, energy, and resources into trying to cope with worries, anxieties, and fears (if coping and other management strategies haven't worked in a lasting way).

- You can choose to leave worries, anxieties, and fears alone and simply experience them as thoughts, sensations, feelings, or painful memories.

- You can choose not to allow anxiety to dictate what you do. As much as you feel like running from intense anxiety, you can learn how to act differently. You can decide to watch anxious feelings and worrisome thoughts and *not* do what they tell you to do.

- You can choose to nurture a kinder and friendlier relationship with yourself and your emotional life rather than react to anxiety as an enemy or unwelcome guest.

- You can decide to move with your anxious discomfort, or any unpleasant thought or emotion, and do something that you really care about.

We know that the solution to anxiety problems is not to fight better or harder. Science and our own work as therapists, researchers, and fellow human beings teach us as much. We also know that the solution doesn't require replacing negative with positive thoughts like you might do when swapping out a worn-out spark plug in your car. None of this really works with anxiety and fear. And yet, many people do struggle. You probably do too.

You may think that you need to win this battle—perhaps by trying harder, struggling more, learning better strategies, gathering new knowledge about anxiety problems from books and social media, finding a new medication, venting, and so on.

But here's the hard truth. Nobody ever wins this kind of battle. We get that this may sound depressing. It may even leave you feeling a bit hopeless. But there's an upside to this hard truth. You don't have to win this battle to get your life back.

What you do need to do is change your relationship with, and response to, your anxious thoughts and feelings. This is how you get out from under the constant oppression of anxiety and fear. You choose to stop fighting. To do that, you'll need to develop your capacity for perspective, or awareness. You cannot change what you don't know or what you're unwilling to look at. This awareness will help you acknowledge anxious thoughts and feelings without becoming them, acting on them, and doing what they say. This will give you freedom to use your precious time on this earth doing what you care deeply about rather than trying to control anxiety.

The prize we're after is your life lived to its fullest!

LEARNING TO BE RIGHT WHERE YOU ARE

Anxiety and fear will pull you into dark places and far from where you are in the moment. These emotions want you to be anywhere else but here and now. This is a problem, because your life is lived in the present moment, and the next, and so on. So, to counter this natural tendency, you'll need to learn how to come back to where you are. We'd like to invite you to practice a simple centering exercise. You could also think of it as a grounding exercise, or as a skillful way to train yourself to be present wherever you are.

This centering practice will help you be right where you are *and* become more consciously aware of what matters to you. This practice will also help you come back to the present in your daily life when anxiety or other painful experiences try hard to pull you out of the moment.

Be mindful that there is no right or wrong way to practice. Just follow along as best you can. All you need to do is get in a comfortable position where you won't be disturbed for five minutes. Remember, you can download the audio file from the workbook website (http://www.newharbinger.com/54476) and then just close your eyes and listen along. You may also use the script below, though we've found that it is better to listen and follow along.

If you'd rather keep your eyes open, you can do that too, but it's best to focus on a spot, say on the floor just in front of you, so you don't get too distracted. The recording ends the exercise with a small chime and tells you when to open your eyes and move on.

EXERCISE: Simple Centering

Go ahead and get in a comfortable position in your chair. Sit upright with your feet flat on the floor, your arms and legs uncrossed, and your hands resting in your lap. Allow your eyes to close gently. Take a couple of gentle breaths—in...and out...in...and out. Notice the sound and feel of your own breath as you breathe in...and out...

Now turn your attention to being just where you are. Notice any sounds that you may hear close to you and then farther away. Notice how you're sitting in your chair, and feel the place where your body touches the chair. What are the sensations there? How does it feel to sit where you sit?

Next, notice the places where your body touches itself, and bring your awareness to the spot where your hands touch your lap or legs. And now, imagine your awareness pouring down over your hips to where your feet touch the floor. How do your feet feel in the position that they are in? Notice too that your feet are firmly grounded to the floor and earth beneath you.

Now gently expand your awareness and just notice sensations in the rest of your body. If you feel any sensations in your body, just notice them and acknowledge their presence. Also notice how they may, by themselves, change or shift from moment to moment. Do not try to change them.

Now let yourself come back to being just where you are, here with this workbook. See if you can feel the investment of yourself here, right now. What are you here for? If you're thinking this sounds strange, just notice that and come back to the sense of integrity here. Be aware of the value that you are serving by being here.

And, see if you can allow yourself to be present with what you are afraid of. Notice any doubts, reservations, fears, and worries. See if you can just notice them, acknowledge their presence, make some space for them, and allow them to be there. You don't need to make them go away or work on them. With each breath, imagine that you are creating more and more space for them, more space for you to be you, right here where you are. Now see if for just a moment you can be present with your values and commitments. Why are you here, working with this workbook? Where do you want to go? What do you want to do with your life?

Then, when you're ready, let go of those thoughts and gradually widen your attention to take in the sounds around you, and slowly open your eyes with the intention to bring this awareness to the present moment and the rest of the day.

Let's take a moment to reflect on your experience with the Simple Centering exercise. What's important here is that you begin to notice your experience and what it teaches you. This will give you a sense of where you are as you begin your journey. So, let's start there.

What showed up for you as you considered your intentions? Why are you here, working with this workbook now to make changes in your life?

_____

_____

What physical sensations, if any, were you able to notice in your body?

_____

_____

List any thoughts that showed up that seemed to pull you out of the exercise (e.g., *I can't con-centrate. This is boring. I'm not doing this right. My mind is racing.*). Be specific, as if you're quoting yourself.

_____

_____

Were you attached to any particular result by doing the practice—like feeling more relaxed, calm, or at peace? If so, note this below.

_____

_____

We encourage you to practice this Simple Centering exercise daily. Find a time and place that's right for you. Over time, this exercise will help you create the space you need to show up to your life and do what you care about.

WHAT IS ACT?

This workbook is based in evidence supporting a revolutionary approach known as *acceptance and commitment therapy* (ACT, pronounced like the word "act"). This pronunciation is important because it summarizes what ACT ultimately stands for: committed ACT*ion*.

Accept—Choose—Take Action

The easiest way to get the gist of ACT is to focus on the three steps that the letters represent: Accept—Choose—Take action. Put another way, ACT is about letting go, showing up to life, and getting yourself moving in directions you want to go. Don't worry if this strikes you as too general or idealistic. We'll get more specific as you move on and practice the exercises. For now, we'll unpack the ACT acronym just a bit to give you a sense of what's to come.

Accept

The idea is to accept what you're already experiencing and cannot control. Acceptance also involves active skills that will help you to respond differently—with kindness, compassion, gentleness, and less engagement—when anxieties, fears, worries, panic, and other sources of emotional and psychological pain show up.

As you learn to open up and drop the rope in the tug-of-war with your anxiety monsters, the need to eliminate or change anxiety and fear washes away, and so does the suffering. You'll also notice that your hands, feet, mind, and mouth will be freed up for other important things in your life. In the process, anxiety will become a smaller part of your larger life.

Choose

ACT will also help you choose a direction for your life. This can be helpful whether you know where you're headed or not. Choosing a direction means identifying what you value in life and what you want your life to stand for. Here, you'll get a chance to discover what's most important to you—what you value—and then make a choice. What kind of child, sibling, student, or friend do you want to be? What types of activities are meaningful to you?

Answering these kinds of questions is about choosing to go forward in directions that are uniquely yours *and* about accepting whatever arises in your mind or body along the way. Are you willing to be open to what your mind and body are doing anyway, fully and without avoiding or trying to escape from it? If the answer is no, you and your life will tend to get smaller while your anxiety grows larger. If the answer is yes, you'll get bigger and your life will expand too. Living well will become your focus rather than living to feel better.

Take Action

Finally, you'll commit to taking steps toward realizing your valued life goals. This part involves action—or doing something—and changing what can be changed. You'll learn how to behave in ways that align with your values. As you work with the material, you'll begin to see that there's a difference between you as a person, your actions, and your thoughts and feelings. We won't be asking you to face your fears in the hope of a better life. Instead, we'll help you cultivate willingness to move with emotional discomfort as you step toward your life goals and dreams.

Each of the three bold steps can feel intimidating, even scary. You may find yourself thinking, *I can't do this now...it's too much...maybe another time.* These thoughts are perfectly okay; it's just your mind doing its thing. Do your best to hold your thoughts lightly. Keep reading. Let the thoughts be what they are, and let your mind do what it does. Allow all thoughts and feelings to come and go as they please.

WHY ACT?

Recall the list of anxiety management and control strategies we covered earlier? On the surface, they appear different from one another, but they're all about one thing—struggle. Let's explore what research can teach us about struggle with emotional and psychological distress:

■ **It increases activity of the sympathetic branch of your nervous system.** This system is the engine that ignites when you feel anxious, angry, or when your life is in danger. It makes you feel ramped up and uncomfortable. Think fight, flight, or freeze.

■ **It worsens memory for important life events. Your ability to remember depends, in part, on what you attend to.** Focusing attention on anxiety and hurt will make anxiety more memorable. It also pulls your attention away from other meaningful activities, so you don't process them fully, and you end up being forgetful.

■ **It's effortful.** It takes lots of energy and effort to push against unpleasant thoughts, feelings, and memories. Think of it as trying to use the palm of your hand to hold back a stream of water gushing out of a garden hose. It doesn't work, and you just end up getting soaked.

■ **It works just well enough in the short term.** This is why people keep doing it—resisting or avoiding anxious thoughts and feelings often will buy you some temporary relief. In the long run, though, it doesn't work. People continue to suffer and pay a price for short-term relief.

■ **It doesn't change the quality of negative thoughts and feelings.** In fact, people tend to feel as bad or worse during and after fighting unpleasant thoughts and feelings. And, on top of that, it's exhausting.

■ **It diminishes your capacity for happiness and joy.** Pleasant and unpleasant emotions and thoughts all flow from the same source. When you try to stop the unpleasant ones, you also block your capacity to feel genuine happiness, joy, and peace.

■ **It pulls you out of your life.** This is the most important finding. People who fight their thoughts and feelings on a regular basis report poorer quality of life, feeling less authentic, having fewer close relationships, and generally feeling limited in what they do. They feel stuck.

Decades of research and wisdom point to one undeniable fact: trying to change anxious thoughts and feelings doesn't work. Period!

This is where ACT comes in, offering a path out of anxiety without the usual struggle and control. Instead, you learn to do the opposite. You change your relationship with your anxious discomfort—especially how you respond in the presence of it—by no longer fighting or resisting it. This is what we mean when we say that ACT is all about allowing yourself to feel what you feel and think what you think while doing what works and is important to you. In essence, ACT combines acceptance with change. You need both to get your life back.

You've probably heard the basic message of ACT in another form—the well-known serenity creed: *Grant me serenity to accept the things I cannot change, courage to change what I can change, and the wisdom to know the difference.*

While this sounds simple, applying it is often challenging. Many people struggle to do what the serenity creed asks. Why? Because most of us simply don't know the difference between what we *can* and *cannot* change. Many more don't know how to accept and live with unpleasant thoughts and feelings. The upshot is that few know how to apply this profound statement to their daily lives. We'll show you how.

When you read this book and do the exercises, you'll learn how to recognize what you can and cannot change. Acceptance and mindfulness practices will help you accept the things you have no control over and cannot change. You'll also learn how to make space for all of your experiences—everything your mind throws at you, what your body does, and your emotional life. With acceptance and compassion, you'll learn how to redirect your focus, so you can use your precious time and energy doing what matters to you. This shift will lead you out of your worries, anxieties, and fears and back into your life.

HOPE AND CHANGE: THE ACT WITH ANXIETY WAY

Before wrapping up this chapter, we'd like to pull together some key elements of this workbook to help you see what you are getting into and what you can expect. We'll do this with some cartoons and a few text prompts. Just imagine that you are the person illustrated in the cartoon.

This image is about what most people want. Notice that you're moving toward what you really care about in this life. You are free, engaging life to its fullest. Wouldn't that be something? But you know this is not how life always works. In fact, if this image were true of the human experience, then there would be no need for therapists, psychiatrists, and coaches. You know that life often offers challenges that make doing what you care about hard.

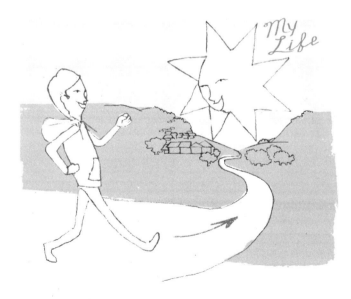

In fact, as you step forward, all kinds of things show up—sometimes unpleasant things.

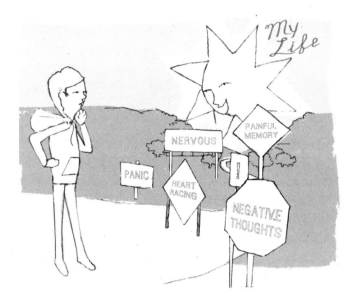

And so you stop.

You think.

You fret, wallow, and stew.

And you do what seems like the most sensible thing to do. You try to get the "bad" stuff out of the way because it seems to stand between you and your life. You're not alone in that. Many people get stuck here.

Notice that as you're trying to get a handle on your discomfort, you stop and have turned your back on your life and where you wanted to go. And your life notices this too: "Huh…what about me?"

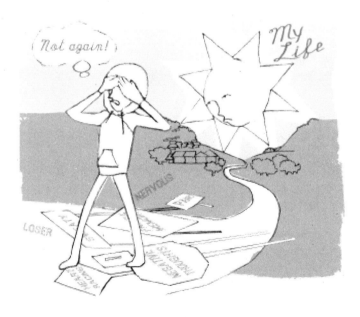

Your life waits as you pour your energies into getting a grip. You try many ways of coping, but nothing seems to work.

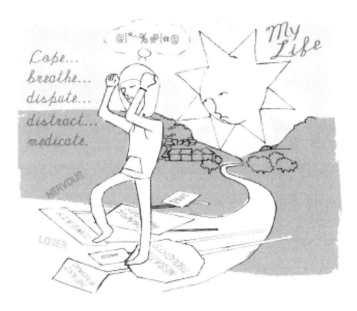

On and on it goes—a scene that has played out countless times. All the while, time is ticking by… ticktock…ticktock. There you are struggling, and your life is waiting, just waiting. And your life becomes sad too, because you're stuck in a battle with anxiety and fear and not living your life.

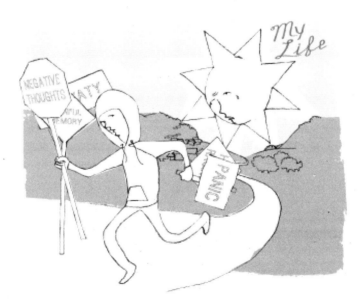

If your go-to coping strategies fail, you may leave the situation. Here, notice where your anxious thoughts and feelings go when you leave. They go with you, right? There's no way to leave anxiety behind. More importantly, leaving is moving you in the opposite direction of where you wanted to go.

You're now left feeling exhausted, frustrated, at your wit's end, head hung low.

And your mind is still at work feeding you more negative news. *Why can't I be normal? Why can't I get a handle on my anxiety and fears? Why can't I be happy like everyone else? Maybe something is wrong with me!*

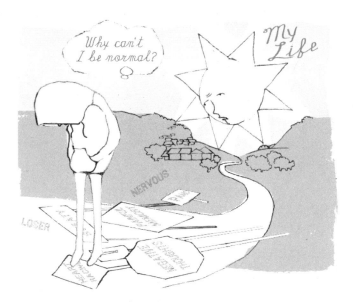

So there you are, stuck, wallowing in this "out of my life" place with pain on top of pain. You feel bad, broken, and without hope. You may even feel sad that you've once again missed out on important things in your life. You might feel cheated, even angry at yourself too. Notice that your life is sadder than before and is still waiting for you.

But then something changes.

Something profound and beautiful happens.

You see what's really going on.

You take stock.

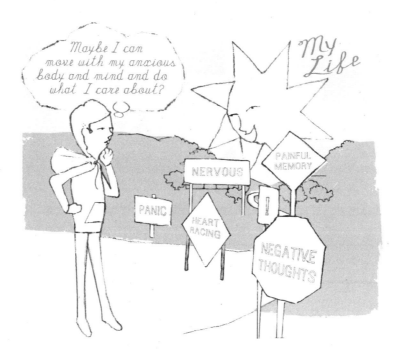

You say, "Enough is enough."

You open up to other possibilities.

Maybe, just maybe, thoughts and feelings are not barriers after all. Maybe they're just part of you. Perhaps you can bring them along as you do what you care about.

Your life seems to like this idea.

So you take a bold and courageous step forward in directions you want to go. As you step, you bring compassion and kindness to whatever shows up inside your mind and body. You're moving. You're headed back into your life and doing what matters to you.

Your life notices right away. Others notice right away. You notice right away.

You commit to doing what you care about with whatever your mind or old history dishes out.

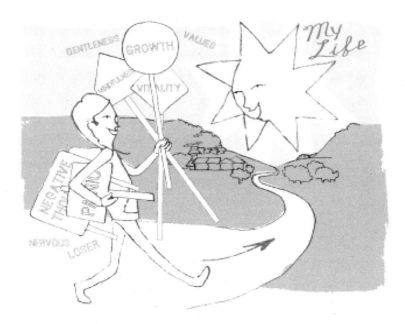

And as you do more of that, your life improves. Your life enjoys spending time with you!

This last illustration sums up the approach we take in this workbook. It also gives you a glimpse of the life-affirming changes you can expect.

Elements in all the preceding scenes will be addressed in this workbook too, except one. We know of no healthy way to stop unpleasant thoughts and feelings from showing up from time to time (see the second cartoon in this section). When you're fully engaged in living your life, you're bound to get all sorts of thoughts, feelings, and bodily sensations. You can't have a life without being willing to experience a full range of thoughts and feelings.

But we'll teach you how to keep your anxious mind and body from standing between you and your life. You'll learn to stop anxiety management that leads you to turn your back on your life.

You'll learn how to stop struggling with your emotional and psychological discomfort. You'll develop skills to be kinder to yourself so that you don't wallow or beat yourself up with more negative judgments and blame. Most importantly, we'll show you how to win the war with your anxiety, not by defeating it but by welcoming it as you engage your life one step at a time.

Living well is how you'll defeat anxiety. It starts by acting on your anxiety differently than you have done before. This is the way to create the conditions for your genuine happiness!

YOUR COMMITMENT TO CHANGE

Commitment is a central component of any effort to change. Are you ready for that commitment and willing to learn another way to approach your worry, anxiety, and fear—and your life?

Answering "yes" means that you're one step closer to taking control over your actions and committing to move yourself in life directions you truly value. If you answered that way, great!

If you answered "no," then stop. Ask yourself, *What's getting in my way?* Look inside yourself first, and then look for barriers in the world around you. Write the barriers down in the space below and be as specific as possible.

_____

_____

_____

_____

_____

_____

Look at your barriers. Take some time with them if you need to do that.

Be mindful that we're not asking you to overcome any barriers. We're only asking if you're willing to learn a different way of relating with your anxieties, fears, and the like. Only you can decide whether the barriers continue to stand between you and getting something different out of your life. When you're 100 percent willing to make this commitment, do it, and do it again and again with each new chapter.

Commitment doesn't mean you have to get everything right. We all experience setbacks and at times slide back into old habits. When that happens, do the best you can.

There will be times when you break one of your commitments. But that doesn't mean you've failed or, worse, that *you* are a failure. Give yourself a break. This is just your mind talking. Beating yourself up for being human is never helpful. In fact, it's a surefire way to feel worse.

Here's why we think commitment is so important: without commitment to action—if you don't complete the exercises—nothing much is going to change in your life. We've touched on this theme already in this chapter, but it's worth repeating the mantra: *If I continue to do what I've always done, then I'm going to get what I've always got.*

Many people attribute this quote to Anthony Robbins and, before him, to Albert Einstein, Henry Ford, Mark Twain, and even Steven Hayes and the developers of ACT. Who coined the phrase isn't important. What is worth looking at is the wisdom it contains for how to change your life for the better. This mantra teaches us that if we want to change the result, then we need to change the way we do things.

Pause for a moment and let this message sink in. What does it mean to you? When you commit to doing something new, can you imagine the possibilities that lie ahead for you? Or, what your life could become? If not, the next exercise will help you get in touch with that.

EXERCISE: Your Life Book of Possibilities

It's impossible to go forward while always looking back, focused on what's wrong with you and your life, or repeating the same old patterns that led you to this place. It's also next to impossible to commit to anything unless you can see it clearly. So, let's shift the perspective and get some clarity.

Take a few moments to pause and allow your eyes to close gently. Bring your awareness to your breath and where you are, right now, at this moment in your life. Simply settle into the now and give yourself permission to just be here. And when you're ready, slowly open your eyes and continue reading.

Hold out your hands in front of you, palms facing up, and imagine that you're holding a book called *Your Life*. This is a book that you know all too well. As you look at this book, you'll notice that several of its pages are already written. They cover the familiar events and experiences you've lived through from the moment you were born, up until now. You see large and small moments, joys, and perhaps enormous hardship and pain. This book also includes your struggles with anxiety and fear. You know the story.

But, as you flip through this book, you may also notice that the story ends abruptly. There's nothing written on the opening page of the new chapter called "Tomorrow." In fact, every page from this moment forward is blank. All you see are pages upon pages of plain white paper.

You may think, *That's strange...maybe I bought a defective book*. But what you're noticing isn't strange at all. In fact, it is exactly the way life works. Your life story from here on out has yet to be written. It's full of possibilities, experiences, and new journeys. Allow yourself to pause again and sink into that truth for a moment. And when you're ready, continue reading.

Now, ask yourself this: *What do I want the next page to say about me and my life?* Will the chapter called "Tomorrow" be just a repeat of yesterday and the days, weeks, and months that came before? If you could put anything down on the next blank page of the book called *Your Life*, what would it be? What do you really want to be about, from this moment forward?

This is the place where your commitment comes in. It needs to be specific, and you need to become consciously aware of it. In the space below, take a moment to jot down what you would like the next page of your life book to say. Be specific. Think in terms of possibilities. Think in terms of what you (and only you) can do. Just write down a few words or sentences that capture the essence of what you'd like to be about and what you'd like to become. What you say here could be as simple as, "I'm going to spend fifteen minutes reading and working with the material in this workbook to change the course of my life." Or, "I'm going to start my day with the Simple Centering exercise I learned about in the introduction."

_____

_____

_____

LIFE-ENHANCEMENT EXERCISES

For this week and those to come, we'll recommend several activities that you can do. We call them life-enhancement exercises because they're about enhancing the depth and quality of your life. We invite you to review them and commit to what you can reasonably do.

For now, we recommend the following activities:

- Commit to doing the Simple Centering exercise.

- Get a sense of your commitment to this workbook and why this is important to you now.

- Make reading and working with this workbook a priority in your life.

THE TAKE-HOME MESSAGE

Change can be scary and liberating at the same time. It involves some risk. Yet the risk of doing more of the same ought to be more frightening. To get something new, all of us need to do something new. It's that simple. And it starts with you making a choice and a commitment to do that. You have much to gain and really nothing to lose.

Preparing Myself for Something New in My Life

Reflections:

- To get something new, I must do something new.

Inquiries:

- Am I ready to choose a new approach with my anxieties, fears, and worries?

- If not, then what's getting in my way?

CHAPTER 2

You Are Not Alone

The truth is that our finest moments are most likely to occur when we are feeling deeply uncomfortable, unhappy, or unfulfilled. For it is only in such moments, propelled by our discomfort, that we are likely to step out of our ruts and start searching for different ways or truer answers.

—M. Scott Peck

Many people suffering with anxiety feel utterly alone. You may feel that way, thinking that nobody understands what it's like to feel the way you feel. In a sense, you're right. Nobody knows your experience better than you. But that doesn't mean you're alone in this either.

As you read this chapter and discover some facts about anxiety, you'll see that countless people all over the world share your fears, struggles, and behavioral tendencies. You'll also see that anxiety problems, including yours, are well recognized and understood. As you learn more, we hope you'll discover that there is hope and you're not so alone!

People with anxiety disorders, and those who experience significant anxiety symptoms, are everywhere. They live in every town, state, and country. Anxiety disorders also affect the rich and the poor alike. In fact, anxiety disorders affect about 33.7 percent of the population at some point in their lifetimes (Bandelow and Michaelis 2015; Kessler et al. 2005).

If that number seems abstract to you, think one-third of the population. That is, one out of three people is someone with an anxiety disorder. But even this may underestimate the extent of anxiety problems, particularly since the COVID-19 pandemic.

Studies show that more people now than before the pandemic are affected by significant anxiety (Vahratian et al. 2021). This amounts to about forty million adults in the United States alone (National Center for Health Statistics, US Census Bureau, Household Pulse Survey 2020–2023), with females outnumbering males two to one. There is also another substantial subgroup who do not have a formal anxiety disorder diagnosis and yet still experience significant anxiety symptoms and poor quality of life.

To bring these numbers home, we'd like you to imagine everyone with an anxiety disorder diagnosis and many others who are dealing with significant but undiagnosed anxiety symptoms. Suppose all of them decided to wear a red hat today. If that were so, you'd have a hard time going about your day without seeing someone with a red hat.

Anxiety disorders tend to be chronic, costly, and debilitating. This means that without some changes on your part, the problems tend to stick around and may worsen over time.

Given the numbers, it's not surprising that anxiety disorders are associated with enormous personal, social, and economic costs. In fact, the global annual direct costs of anxiety disorders is about $6.5 trillion, or the budget of a small country (Arikian and Gorman 2001; Konnopka and König 2020). We should add that this figure does not include the many hidden costs of anxiety disorders and untreated anxiety symptoms. These hidden costs can be summarized in four words—reduced quality of life.

PAUSE AND GET CENTERED

Before we get into the meat of this chapter, we'd like to slow things down a bit and invite you to do another centering exercise. It'll take about five minutes.

As before, be mindful that there's no right or wrong way to do this exercise. Just follow along as well as you can. If you'd rather keep your eyes open, it's best to focus on a spot, say on the floor just in front of you, so you don't get too distracted. We'll end the exercise with a small chime and tell you when to open your eyes and move on.

EXERCISE: Centering into Your Heart

Get in a comfortable position in your chair. Sit upright with your feet flat on the floor, your arms and legs uncrossed, and your hands resting in your lap. Allow your eyes to close gently. Take a couple of gentle breaths—in...and out...in...and out. As you're doing so, notice the sound and feel of your own breath.

Now turn your attention to being just where you are. Notice any sounds that you may hear close to you and then farther away. Notice how you are sitting in your chair. What are the sensations there?

Next, notice the places where your body touches itself, and bring your awareness to the spot where your hands touch your lap or legs. And now imagine your awareness pouring down over your hips to where your feet touch the floor. How do your feet feel in the position that they are in? Notice that your feet are firmly grounded to the floor and earth beneath you.

Now gently expand your awareness and just notice sensations in the rest of your body. If you feel any sensations in your body, notice them and acknowledge their presence. Also notice how they may, by themselves, change or shift from moment to moment. Don't try to change them.

When you're ready, allow your awareness to drift back, ever so slowly and gently, to your breath, and just be here, right where you are. Notice that your breath is still with you, and along with it, the rising and falling of your chest and belly as you breathe in...and out. Imagine that with each breath in, you are creating more and more space inside of you to just be here. Let each breath expand your heart, creating more space within you as you breathe in...and then slowly out. Notice the space within you growing even just a little bit with each inhale you take, and then softening with each exhale.

Now, bring your awareness to that space within you, just about in your center in the middle of your chest. Imagine settling your awareness in that special space close to your heart, however large or small it may be. Let your awareness settle and rest easily there. Breathe gently and sense your breath going into that space around your heart.

And as your awareness settles in that heart space, we'd like to invite you to get in touch with your intentions. Why are you here? What do you want to be about? What do you want to become? And breathe. Soften to what shows up for you.

As we conclude this practice, we'd like to invite you to hold your intentions lightly, as you might hold a small butterfly or a tiny baby in your arms. Don't let go. Just see if you can bring lightness, care, and gentleness to yourself and the intentions you hold dear.

And then, when you're ready, go ahead and take two deep cleansing breaths by filling your lungs fully, and then slowly releasing the air. Repeat that once again, and then slowly open your eyes while gently holding your intentions close to your heart as you go about your day.

WHAT IS THE NATURE OF ANXIETY AND FEAR?

All humans are born with the capacity to experience anxiety and fear. If you're reading this book, then you likely think you have "too much of it." You've probably educated yourself a bit about the nature of anxiety and fear too.

Here, our intention is to add a bit to what you may know. And we'd like to offer you a slightly different perspective.

Before we continue, take a moment to jot down what you think are three critical differences between "normal" and "abnormal" anxiety and fear. For instance, you might think that normal anxiety is less intense compared with abnormal anxiety.

- Normal anxiety/fear is _____ compared with abnormal anxiety/fear.

- Normal anxiety/fear is _____ compared with abnormal anxiety/fear.

- Normal anxiety/fear is _____ compared with abnormal anxiety/fear.

Hold your ideas lightly as you read on. We'll start with the most basic and primitive of all emotions—fear.

Fear: The Present-Focused Basic Emotion

Fear is an intensely felt alarm response. It arises in a flash and often in response to real or perceived threats in the world around you. But you may also be afraid of physical sensations, thoughts, and images that show up inside you.

Fear has been essential for survival throughout human history, and it still serves an important function today. Its primary job is to activate you when your safety or health is threatened. In fact, the primary purpose of fear is to keep you safe and alive. In moments of genuine danger, fear mobilizes your resources and motivates you to take action to protect yourself.

Fear also triggers a cascade of responses in both your brain and body, propelling you into a heightened state of alertness. Your senses become sharper, enabling you to be more attuned to your surroundings and quickly identify potential threats (Barlow 2004).

Various bodily systems are activated too. For instance, you may experience rapid heartbeat, breathlessness, smothering sensations, or increased blood pressure; you may feel hot, sick to your stomach, dizzy, or you may break out in a sweat. You may even feel as though you're about to pass out.

All this activity may leave you with a feeling of heightened energy—the adrenaline rush. These bodily changes, though brief, are necessary to help you take swift action when faced with threat or danger. In the moment, they propel you to fight, flee, or freeze.

Some of these actions are so automatic and hardwired that you don't need to learn them. You just react without conscious thought. As an example, do you remember a time when someone startled you by jumping out from behind a door, causing your heart to race and your body to tense up? This is what we mean by an automatic reaction. Fear happens.

But you can also learn to respond with fear, often with the help of language. Consider how hearing someone shout "Get out—the building is on fire!" can trigger a fearful response, even if you don't see the fire yourself. Language allows people to evoke fear in themselves and other people without needing to confront the source of threat directly. This piece highlights the power of words to elicit strong emotional reactions.

Anxiety: The Future-Focused Emotion

Anxiety, unlike fear, is a future-oriented mood state. This means you're anxious about something yet to happen. Perhaps it's a trip, or a health checkup. Maybe it's an exam, or a job evaluation. Anything in your future is a potential target for anxiety.

When you're feeling anxious, you may notice apprehension or a sense of foreboding, worry, and muscle tension. You may also feel keyed up and on edge. Unlike fear, the physical manifestations of anxiety tend to be much less pronounced and dramatic. Yet anxiety and worry can last much longer than fear, often waxing and waning for days, weeks, months, or even years. This is possible, in part, because anxiety is fueled by thoughts and mental images your mind conjures about future events, not what's actually happening in the moment.

As uncomfortable as anxiety can be, it's important to be mindful that you still need the capacity to experience anxiety. Why? Because it can help motivate you to get things done and can keep you out of harm's way.

In fact, it would be maladaptive not to worry about possible future events that could truly threaten your health and welfare. We know that anxiety and worry can help motivate you to plan and prepare for future challenges. For instance, creating an action plan in case of a house fire is a practical and useful response to a potential danger.

EXERCISE: Is There a Difference Between Anxiety and Fear?

Read each item and then circle (A) if you think the event would mostly likely cause anxiety or (F) if you think the event would bring on fear.

• Seeing a bear in the woods	A F	• Possibility of seeing a bear in the woods A F
• Being mugged in the city	A F	• Chance of being mugged in the future A F
• A car almost hitting you	A F	• Possibility of getting hit by a car A F
• Suffering a serious injury	A F	• Chance of being seriously injured A F
• Being in a house fire	A F	• Possibility of your house burning A F

Notice that all the situations in the left column are present focused, whereas those in the right column are future focused, which means you should have all Fs in the left column and all As in the right column. This activity points to the critical difference between fear and anxiety.

People are typically anxious about something that may happen in the future, whereas fear is a reaction to what is or could be happening in the moment. As an example, you might experience anxiety about the possibility of being in an earthquake and living through the aftermath, but fear would be your experience when the earth is shaking beneath you.

In summary, behaviors most closely linked with anxiety have to do with what you think and say to yourself (worrying, ruminating over something, even making plans), whereas behaviors most closely associated with fear involve overt actions (running, fighting, taking cover, freezing). If it helps, you can think of the difference this way: fear involves little thought; anxiety needs big thought.

What About Your Fear and Anxiety?

The next exercise invites you to consider how your fear and anxiety may have been helpful to you. To get started, we'd like you to reflect on a recent or significant experience where you felt fear and this feeling ended up being beneficial to you. We'll do the same with anxiety in a bit.

By "beneficial," we mean a situation where you were suddenly faced with real danger—perhaps a car suddenly swerving into your lane or a person or animal that threatened to harm you. Recall an example that was a big deal for you—where experiencing fear and doing something to save yourself (or someone else) made a real difference, perhaps even saved your own or someone else's life. Here, we're not asking you to recall a significant trauma. Stick with an example you're willing to work with.

This activity may be difficult, because you probably see your anxiety and fear as unwelcome intruders. You may not be in a place where you can see your anxieties and fears as assets, or even as friends or allies. That's perfectly okay for now.

Just give yourself some time to do this exercise. See if you can put the idea that worry, anxiety, and fear are bad to the side for a moment as you think about at least one example from your life where fear and anxiety were helpful for you.

Doing this brief exercise will be useful later when we'll help you figure out when acting on fear and anxiety is helpful versus when it's not helpful, and only makes matters worse.

EXERCISE: Are Fear and Worry Sometimes Useful?

On the lines below, briefly describe the threatening or dangerous event, your response, and how your response was useful. The point is to look at how fear mobilized you to do something for your own safety and welfare (or that of others).

What was the threatening or dangerous event?

_____

What was your response (thoughts, physical sensations, feelings, actions)?

_____

How was your fear response useful in the moment?

_____

Now recall a situation or event where being anxious and worrying about a possible negative event or outcome helped you make a plan, where having a plan and acting on it was somehow useful to you. On the lines below, briefly describe the event, your response, and how your response was useful.

What was the potential problem you were anxious or worried about?

_____

What was your response (thoughts, physical sensations, feelings, actions)?

_____

How was your anxiety response useful in this situation?

_____

It's crucial to recognize that fear and worry have been valuable tools for you in the past and will likely continue to be in the future. Keep this in mind as you work through this book. Consider jotting down a reminder: "I need the capacity to experience worry, anxiety, and fear, just like I need air to breathe, water to drink, and food to eat."

This doesn't mean that you ought to be anxious 24/7. We understand that you may feel like anxiety is with you all the time. You may also feel that your worry, anxiety, and fear are more harmful than helpful. They happen too often or too intensely. They show up when you're at no risk of being harmed. Your worries may seem like they stretch to infinity. Your thoughts are too disturbing and almost impossible to turn off.

Your struggles with anxiety have likely disrupted your life, perhaps even driving you to seek help through this book. This interference with daily living is a crucial indicator that professionals use to distinguish between adaptive anxiety and an anxiety disorder.

Let's have a closer look at how this applies to you.

IDENTIFYING YOUR TYPE OF ANXIETY "PROBLEM"

Self-help books written for people with anxiety-related concerns typically focus too much on describing various types of anxiety problems and helping people diagnose themselves. We don't want to lead you down this path because we don't think it's helpful.

When you label yourself with a diagnosis, you're telling yourself you have something that's painful, undesirable, and self-limiting. This is not helpful if the point is to break free from anxiety and live your life.

Labels are hard to shake once applied and can even become a self-fulfilling prophecy—something you become. It would be better to think of the symptoms of your anxiety problem as descriptions of difficulties you are experiencing now. They do not define you. You can change. Your life can change. What you need to learn is how to accept what needs to be accepted and change what can be changed.

Your most important task is to identify the root of what turns your fear, anxiety, worry, trauma, or obsessions into a life-shattering problem. To get there, you need to be clear about what it is that you've been struggling with for so long. This kind of clarity has another purpose too. We've found that people do better with treatment when they focus their efforts on their most vexing concerns. By concentrating on your most challenging issues, you may find that other related concerns also start to improve.

In the following sections, you'll find descriptions of the major anxiety disorders, symptoms, and related problems based, in part, on how the American Psychiatric Association (2022) defines them. Be mindful that we do not agree with the recent decision by the psychiatric community to move obsessive-compulsive disorder and post-traumatic stress disorder into their own unique categories. In our view, the root of the problems with obsessions, compulsive behaviors, and a traumatic past are the same as anxiety-related concerns. You'll see why in a moment.

You'll also get a chance to read about real people who have struggled with anxiety problems. We've kept their stories brief and have gone to great lengths to protect their identities. You may see some of yourself in their stories. As you read on, look for the commonalities among the different stories. See if you can find the golden thread that binds all anxiety problems together.

Panic Attacks

A panic attack is a sudden rush of fear. It's accompanied by intense physical sensations, a strong urge to escape or get away from the situation or place where those sensations occur, and a sense of impending doom—the feeling that something bad is about to happen.

Below is a list of experiences that define a panic attack. Check (✓) anything that you experience when you have a panic attack:

☐ Pounding or racing heart

☐ Chest pain or discomfort

- ☐ Shortness of breath or smothering sensations

- ☐ Trembling or shaking

- ☐ Feeling of choking

- ☐ Sweating

- ☐ Dizziness, unsteady feeling, or faintness

- ☐ Nausea or abdominal distress

- ☐ Feeling you or your surroundings are strange or unreal

- ☐ Numbness or tingling in face, hands, or legs

- ☐ Hot flashes or chills

- ☐ Fear of losing control or "going crazy"

- ☐ Fear of dying (e.g., fear of having a heart attack)

Panic attacks often seem to show up out of nowhere when you least expect it. Though we know that most panic attacks are triggered by something, when you're in the middle of one, the triggers aren't obvious. They're also called "false alarms" for this reason. The lack of obvious triggers can heighten fear associated with panic attacks, as they appear senseless and devoid of any useful purpose.

We know from many research studies that panic attacks are common. About ten to thirty-three people out of one hundred will have at least one panic attack over a twelve-month period (Barlow 2004). Stress in your life can certainly make panic attacks more likely, but panic attacks can happen during periods of calm too. They can even show up when you're asleep, jarring you awake.

Take the case of Alice, a thirty-one-year-old office clerk and a single mother of two young children. Her first panic attack happened during a stressful day at work.

■ Alice's Story

The company where I work laid off a bunch of people to cut costs. With not as many people in the office, I had to pick up the slack and do the job of two people. I was burning the candle at both ends and felt like I was neglecting my kids. The added workload and longer hours really stressed me out. I clearly remember my first panic attack. I was at work and the boss was riding me about missing invoices for a building contract. That's when I lost it. I remember feeling my heart pounding and a strange tightness in my chest. I couldn't catch my breath either. The room seemed to be spinning and I couldn't keep my focus. I remember thinking, This is it… I'm having a heart attack and am going to die. Who would take care of my little ones? My *boss called 911 and they took me by ambulance to the emergency room. After a bunch of tests, the doctors told me that my heart was fine. That news was comforting, but I still had no idea what happened to me that day. A week or so later, I had another attack at home just before going to bed. I've had many more since. Some attacks happen for no reason, but others seem to start with a tingling sensation in my chest right around my heart. I have since taken a leave of absence from work because I'm afraid of having another attack and making a fool of myself. Now I'm having a hard time making ends meet and caring for my kids.*

How Panic Attacks May Turn into Panic Disorder

Having many unexpected panic attacks without an obvious trigger or cause is one of the official standards used by mental health professionals when diagnosing panic disorder, yet this isn't the whole story. Even if you've had many panic attacks and continue to have them as often as once a month, several times a week, or every day, it doesn't mean you have panic disorder.

A diagnosis of panic disorder requires that you also worry about when the next attack will strike or the possible consequences of an attack. For instance, you might worry that you'll die, lose control, faint, go crazy, vomit, or have diarrhea. You may even think that you'll humiliate yourself, lose your job, or end up being hospitalized. Getting hooked on these thoughts can certainly make things worse, but they're not the most important feature of panic disorder.

The main difference between panic and panic disorder has to do with a change in your behavior. As we saw with Alice, you start doing things to avoid or prevent experiencing panic and stop doing things that are important to you. The result? Your life becomes smaller.

We've summarized some of the more common behavioral changes for you below (Antony and McCabe 2004). As you'll see, the behaviors look different, but underneath, they're quite similar—they all serve to make people feel safe (or at least safer) from panic. Check (✔) all behaviors in the list that you engage in to manage your panic:

☐ Sitting near exits at the movies or in a restaurant

☐ Checking where the closest exit is when visiting a shopping mall

☐ Carrying medication, money, cell phone, pager, water, or other safety items

☐ Avoiding activities (e.g., exercise, sex, thriller movies) that trigger physical arousal

☐ Drinking alcohol or using other drugs

☐ Avoiding caffeine, alcohol, or other substances (e.g., MSG, spicy foods)

☐ Frequently checking your pulse or blood pressure

☐ Distracting yourself from the panic experience (for instance, reading a book, watching TV, scrolling through social media)

☐ Insisting on being accompanied when leaving the house

☐ Always needing to know the whereabouts of your spouse, partner, or "safe" person

Some people with panic disorder don't avoid situations where panic attacks may occur. With courage and determination, they refuse to let panic attacks dictate what they do. Most people with panic disorder, however, develop some degree of agoraphobia over time, which simply means they avoid places or events where panic attacks might happen. These are often places where escape is difficult, where help may not be readily available if needed, and where there's a sense of feeling confined or trapped.

Here are some of the most common situations people avoid. Again, check (✓) all situations in the list that you avoid so you won't have a panic attack:

☐ Crowded public places (e.g., supermarkets, theaters, malls, sports events)

☐ Enclosed and confined places (e.g., tunnels, bridges, small rooms, elevators, airplanes, subways, buses, hair salons, waiting in line or at traffic lights)

☐ Driving (especially on highways and bridges, in bad traffic, and over long distances)

☐ Being away from home (such as having a safe distance around your home beyond which you find it difficult to travel, or feeling like you can't leave your home)

☐ Being alone (at home or in any of the situations listed above)

Let's look at how some of this played out with Jack, a forty-nine-year-old accountant. His frequent panic attacks have morphed into panic disorder. He not only worries about future attacks but also has changed his behavior to avoid having them. As you'll see, Jack has some agoraphobic avoidance, as he avoids places where panic may attack.

■ *Jack's Story*

I had my first panic attack about twenty years ago. I was driving on the highway to my first real job at an accounting firm. During that drive, I began to tremble and shake. Within minutes, I broke out in a cold sweat and felt like I couldn't breathe. Then, the numbness started in my hands, and I felt like I couldn't feel the steering wheel. I really thought I was going to die or get in an accident. So, I pulled over and just sat there. I eventually calmed down, called my firm to say I was taking a sick day, and then made my way back home. Since then, I've stopped driving anywhere outside a seven-mile radius from my home. Highways are out. Leaving the house is rare. Though my firm wanted me back in the office, I told them I couldn't get there on my own. Initially, they allowed me to work remotely, but I couldn't juggle all the demands, and so quit and am now on disability. My wife has been a huge support, but I feel badly for her. Our finances are extremely tight. We don't go out because I am too scared to go out. She has family about forty miles from our house, but I don't feel comfortable going that far outside my safe zone or with her leaving to visit them without me. Since that infamous drive, I have had several panic attacks and am sick of living in a shell. I also worry about my marriage. How much more will my wife take? I get that I am dealing with agoraphobia, but my problems have become her problems. My limitations have become her limitations.

Specific Phobias

Just about everyone has something that they're afraid of. You probably do too. But specific phobias are more than just an extreme fear of something. They also involve excessive avoidance. When you struggle with a specific phobia, you experience a strong urge to avoid the feared object or situation. Many are successful at doing just that, but for others the avoidance can be quite costly.

Large surveys teach us that about 13 percent of the population will struggle with a specific phobia during their lifetime (Kessler et al. 2005). The most common specific phobias (in descending order) are fear of animals, heights, closed spaces, blood and injuries, storms and lightning, and flying.

Many people with specific phobias also experience an alarm reaction that is virtually identical to a panic attack. Unlike panic disorder, the alarm response in specific phobias is triggered by obvious cues. This is also true for phobias of blood, injections, or injuries, except that the fear is followed by a sudden drop in blood pressure, leaving people feeling faint or losing consciousness for a bit.

People with specific phobias also recognize that their fear is excessive or unreasonable. But this awareness has no impact on the fear itself or the urge to run from and avoid feared objects. It also does little to help them control or reduce the unpleasant emotional discomfort that's triggered by feared objects or situations.

Look at the list below and check (✔) all items that give you an intense panic-like response when you encounter them:

☐ Situations (e.g., heights, closed spaces, dentists, elevators, airplanes or flying)

☐ Animals (e.g., snakes, rats, spiders, dogs)

☐ Natural environment (e.g., heights, storms, lightning, water)

☐ Illness or bodily harm (e.g., diseases, injuries)

☐ Sight of blood or needles

☐ Other (e.g., choking, eating certain foods, clowns, vomiting)

Most people with specific phobias never seek treatment. They simply avoid the feared object. This is easy to do when the feared object is clearly known or unlikely to be encountered. So, if you have a shark phobia and live in Idaho, it's highly unlikely that you'll have much difficulty with this phobia. There's no chance of running into a shark in Idaho (other than in movies or on TV). As a result, this phobia would not interfere with daily life.

At times, avoidance may appear successful but it comes at a high personal cost. For instance, we once worked with an Australian family who used to enjoy weekends on a beautiful island just offshore. The family stopped going because the mother had a shark phobia. She couldn't stand the thought of sharks swimming underneath the ferryboat during the crossing.

Here, this woman's life was asking her to make a choice between two options. She could either choose to spend time with her family in a beautiful setting and allow herself to feel the fear while getting there, or she could stay at home without fear and miss out on a fun time with her family. The answer was obvious to her—family. Coming to terms with that choice made a real difference in her life. But getting there wasn't easy.

Avery, a thirty-five-year-old with a lifelong phobia of worms, also had to face some tough choices. As you'll see, her fear and avoidance was controlling her and limiting her life.

■ Avery's Story

I have always loved the changing seasons. Well, except for the start of spring. When the ground thaws, the worms come out. I know it doesn't make sense, but I'm terrified of worms. They're ugly, and I feel like they're everywhere. On the sidewalks, the roads, and even the walkway to my front door. I like to walk to work for exercise, but in the spring, this walk is unbearable. I am constantly looking down trying to avoid stepping on one of them. All the while I am gagging and feel like I'm about to vomit. I've arrived at work more than once with tears streaming down my face. It's gotten so bad that I've asked my fiancé to drive me to work and to clear a worm-free path from the door to the car. I've also stopped doing my daily walks because the anxiety and disgust is so intense. Just thinking about them gets my pulse racing. When I see them or, even worse, step on one of them, I hyperventilate and want to puke. I do everything I can to avoid going outside in early spring.

Avery eventually got help and began using some of the ideas and skills we describe in this book. She became determined to not let her fear and avoidance of worms control her life. She never ended up liking worms, but she learned not to let her fear get in the way of what she wanted to do.

Social Anxiety Disorder

Feeling anxious, self-conscious, or awkward in social situations is common, but social anxiety disorder is more than that. It's also not the same as just being shy or introverted.

Social anxiety is an intense fear of embarrassment or humiliation. Usually, this fear shows up when you're exposed to the possibility that other people may judge or criticize you. For some, social anxiety is limited to situations where you must perform or speak in front of others. You may fear that you'll say or do something stupid and then be judged harshly for it. You may also worry that people can detect your social anxiety.

Social anxiety disorder is also more than extreme anxiety in social situations or fearing embarrassment, judgment by others, or humiliation. People suffering from social anxiety disorder avoid social situations to avoid feeling anxious. As you might imagine, trying to avoid interactions with other people is extremely hard to do without significant costs.

It might surprise you to learn that social anxiety ranks number one of all the anxiety disorders globally, with about 12 percent of the US population suffering from it at some point during their lives (Stein et al. 2017). Let's take a closer look.

Below is a list of common social fears that lead people to avoid social situations. You'll see that fear of public speaking tops the list. It's the most common trigger for social anxiety and a concern shared by many. Check (✓) all of the social fears that apply to you:

- ☐ Fear of public speaking

- ☐ Fear of blushing in public

- ☐ Fear of eating or drinking in public, including choking or spilling food

- ☐ Fear of writing or signing documents when others are present (e.g., at grocery checkout)

- ☐ Fear of being watched (e.g., at work, working out, shopping, dining out)

- ☐ Fear of crowds

- ☐ Fear of using public toilets

- ☐ Fear of going to parties or social gatherings

- ☐ Fear of confrontation (e.g., expressing disagreement, disapproval, your opinions)

- ☐ Fear of meeting strangers

- ☐ Fear of performing

Some people with social anxiety also experience panic attacks. Mostly, these panic attacks are related to a specific type of social situation or being embarrassed and humiliated rather than being confined or trapped. If you experience social anxiety, you may also have some of the following signs and symptoms. Check (✓) all that apply to you.

- ☐ Blush, sweat, or tremble

☐ Have a rapid heart rate

☐ Feel your "mind going blank" or feel nauseous or queasy

☐ Have a rigid body posture or speak with an overly soft voice

☐ Find it difficult to make eye contact, be around people you don't know, or talk to people in social situations, even when you want to

☐ Feel self-consciousness or fear that people will judge you negatively

☐ Avoid places where there are other people

More than 90 percent of all people diagnosed with social anxiety fear and avoid more than one social activity (Barlow 2004). But 10 percent do not avoid social situations, even while experiencing intense anxiety around people. In fact, performers (such as stage actors) and people whose jobs require them to speak and interact with people often do their work with their social anxiety. We'll return to that strategy in chapter 8.

For now, let's take a look at Carl, a thirty-one-year-old struggling with social anxiety. As you read Carl's story, see if you can detect how he's not only distressed in social situations but also doing whatever he can to avoid and get rid of that distress.

■ *Carl's Story*

My parents and older brothers were always the outgoing ones. Me, I was the odd duck. Growing up, I was always a bit shy and an introvert. These qualities made me an easy target for the bullies throughout my school years. Being overweight and uncoordinated for my age didn't help either. I got teased in class, outside of class, and even in front of teachers. They'd call me ugly, stupid, faggot, wimp, and loser. Over time, most of the other kids started avoiding me, and I lost what few friends I had. Nobody ever pulled me aside to tell me that all the stories and name-calling weren't true. The teachers did nothing to stop it either. I tried to explain what was going on to my parents, but they didn't understand and brushed it off. These early experiences left a lasting scar on me. My self-worth and confidence took a huge hit. I began to think of myself as the ugly, fat, unlovable loser who nobody would want to be around. By then I was also heavily into smoking weed and other drugs—anything that would dull the anxiety, shame, and isolation I felt. When I went off to college, things got better for a bit. I could do large classes and crowds of students, no problem. But I also had no close friends, because I was too anxious to be exposed to ridicule and harassment. No dating either. I believed, and still do, that people are always judging me, even when they aren't around me. I lived alone, went home on weekends, and just went to class and studied. I ended up with a degree in physics. My parents suggested that I consider becoming a physics teacher, but the thought of constant interactions with other teachers, staff, and students and their parents terrified me. So I opted for a less challenging, lower-paying job as a hotel reservations clerk. Much of the time I don't have to interact with anyone in person. It's all done through text or online chat. Still, I'm lonely and wish I could develop friendships and even have a romantic partner someday. But I can't shake the anxiety and fear I feel around people.

Obsessive-Compulsive Disorder

When people say things like "they're so OC" or "I'm so OC," they're usually reacting to a person being excessively neat, tidy, orderly, organized, and rule following. But this is not obsessive-compulsive disorder (OCD). People with OCD struggle with unwanted intrusive thoughts that generate a good deal of anxiety and fear. They also struggle with mental or behavioral compulsions that they have a hard time resisting. Let's take a closer look.

Obsessions are recurring and persistent thoughts, impulses, or images that bring on intense anxiety. Examples include images or thoughts of being contaminated with dirt or germs, causing harm to self or others, losing control, forgetting or making mistakes like leaving the door unlocked, and forbidden or taboo thoughts about sex, religion, or harming loved ones.

People often experience these thoughts or images as intrusive, unreasonable, and distressing. Not surprisingly, people with OCD do not want to think about the obsessions and try to resist them. Obsessions can also trigger full-blown panic attacks. But unlike panic disorder, the fear in OCD centers around thoughts or images rather than bodily sensations or fear of panic itself.

Here's a list of some common obsessions. Check (✔) all that apply to you:

☐ Thoughts that you might harm yourself or others

☐ Violent or horrific images

☐ Fear of blurting out obscenities or insults

☐ Fear of stealing things

☐ Fear of being responsible for something terrible happening (e.g., fire, burglary)

☐ Sexual thoughts, images, or urges

☐ Fear of acting on unwanted "forbidden" impulses (incest, homosexuality, aggressive or sexual acts)

☐ Concern with sacrilege and blasphemy, right and wrong, sin, or morality

☐ Concern that someone will have an accident unless things are in the right place

- ☐ Fear of saying certain things because you believe they might come true if you say them

- ☐ Fear of losing things

- ☐ Intrusive nonviolent images, nonsense sounds, words, or music

- ☐ Concerns about dirt, germs, or bodily waste or secretions (e.g., urine, feces, saliva)

- ☐ Concern about getting ill from possible contaminants

- ☐ Concern about environmental contaminants (e.g., asbestos, radiation, toxic waste)

- ☐ Excessive concern with household items (e.g., cleansers, solvents)

- ☐ Excessive concern about animals (such as insects)

As the next list highlights, compulsions are repeated, ritualistic behaviors (for example, checking, hand washing) or mental acts (such as counting, praying). Their purpose is to reduce anxiety and suppress or neutralize the disturbing intrusive thoughts or images. In addition, compulsions offer temporary certainty in response to the uncertainty generated by obsessions. So, if you think, *I might have germs that could kill me*, you may then engage in excessive hand washing to prevent your own demise. But as certainty is only temporary, you get caught up in a cycle of executing compulsions to quiet obsessions.

Attending to obsessions and ritualizing is time consuming. It also puts so many constraints on life that people can literally run out of time to do what they need to do. The OCD cycle also interferes with daily routines and social functioning. In extreme cases, hospitalization may be needed to break the cycle.

Here's a partial list of common compulsions. Check (✓) all behaviors that seem to apply to you:

- ☐ Excessive or ritualized cleaning (e.g., hand washing, bathing, tooth brushing, grooming, toilet routine)

- ☐ Excessive cleaning of household items or other inanimate objects

- ☐ Checking locks, stove, appliances, and so on

- ☐ Checking that you did not/will not harm others or yourself

- ☐ Checking that nothing terrible did/will happen

- ☐ Checking that you didn't make a mistake

- ☐ Needing to repeat routine activities (e.g., jogging, going in or out of a door or getting up or down from a chair, brushing your teeth, rereading, rewriting)

- ☐ Compulsively collecting or not being able to get rid of useless objects (e.g., junk mail, old newspapers, garbage, and other objects such as ear swabs, wrappers)

☐ Performing mental rituals (other than checking or counting, such as repeating a mantra or prayer)

☐ Excessive list making

☐ Needing to tell, ask, or confess, or touch, tap, rub, or blink

☐ Ritualized eating behaviors

☐ Engaging in superstitious behaviors (such as carrying something for good luck)

☐ Compulsive hair pulling (top of head, eyelashes, eyebrows)

With OCD, you may realize that your obsessions and compulsions are excessive and unreasonable. You've likely tried to ignore or stop them. But that only increases your distress and anxiety. So, you feel driven to perform compulsive acts, chasing relief that never lasts.

The problem is that rituals reduce anxiety briefly, and then anxiety and tension come right back. The same is true of thoughts that trigger anxiety in the first place. In fact, there's solid evidence showing that trying to ignore or suppress unwanted thoughts and images backfires. Instead of lasting relief, you get more of the very thoughts and images that you don't want to have (Wang, Hagger, and Chatzisarantis 2020). This process keeps the vicious cycle going with OCD, as Nathan knew all too well.

Nathan is a twenty-eight-year-old postal worker who feels completely controlled by an endless cycle of recurring obsessions, anxiety, and compulsive counting and repetition.

■ Nathan's Story

When I was around six, I remember a friend telling me that if you think a bad thought, you must do something to cancel it out or else something bad is going to happen. I took that and spun it completely out of control. When my parents went out on date nights, I would freak out thinking that they're gonna die and never come back unless I did something to prevent that outcome. It began with arranging my toy soldiers in triangles—perfect groups of three. Initially I believed that was enough to keep my parents safe, but it expanded to chores, like emptying the dishwasher. If I didn't do it exactly in five minutes, I was sure my mom was going to die. So I kept a timer close by, and sometimes it would take me several tries before I hit the five-minute mark. Getting caught up in rituals has continued as an adult. In my job, I sort a lot of mail. But it takes me hours to do it, because I feel I must read the recipient address on each envelop three times. Why three? I think I read somewhere that the number three is related to Jupiter— the planet of good fortune. So, I think that by rereading addresses, I am preventing catastrophes and bringing people good luck when they get their mail. It also takes me forever to get dressed. If I put on clothes and think about something bad, I have to take them off and put them back on three times. If I am grocery shopping and think about death, I will buy three of whatever item is close by, even if I don't need it. I have wasted so much money and food because of this. A lot of my thoughts are about death and injury, particularly family, but it could involve anyone. It's gotten to the point where I am chronically late for work and other appointments, and my boss has warned me to pick up the pace or I'll lose my job.

Post-Traumatic Stress Disorder

In your lifetime, it's likely that you'll be exposed to a traumatic event. In fact, estimates suggest that between 70 and 90 percent of the population will witness or experience a traumatic event at some point in their lifetime (Benjet et al. 2016; Goldstein et al. 2016). Of these, nearly one-third will be exposed to four or more traumatic events. That's a lot of people.

Although there's still some debate about what qualifies as trauma, these events are generally thought to be experiences that would produce intense fear, terror, and feelings of helplessness in just about anyone. These include being the victim of a violent crime (such as rape, assault, or abuse as an adult or child), witnessing death or serious injury, combat situations (for instance, wounding of self and others, committing or witnessing atrocities), natural disasters (such as earthquakes, tornadoes, floods), and accidents (such as car or plane crashes or fires).

Going through a trauma can be enormously challenging, but it doesn't mean you'll automatically develop post-traumatic stress disorder (PTSD). In fact, only about six out of every hundred people with a trauma history will go on to struggle with PTSD at some point in their lives (Goldstein et al. 2016). Women, in turn, are twice as likely to develop PTSD than men. Here, it's believed that this sex difference is due, in part, to women being more likely to be exposed to forms of interpersonal violence such as rape, physical assault, and abuse.

It's important to be mindful that most people who go through a traumatic event will not develop PTSD. In fact, research with trauma survivors shows that about 25 percent of those who were caught in the buildings after the 9/11 attack developed PTSD. The rest did not. And even if you do develop PTSD, research shows that you're likely to recover with appropriate treatment.

People suffering from PTSD may notice several unpleasant changes a month or more after the traumatic event. Many of these changes affect how people experience themselves and their world. For instance, before being exposed to trauma, you may have felt that the world was generally safe. At that time, you may have been able to feel a range of emotions, and especially love for people and experiences you care about.

But after the trauma, things change. You may now see the world as a dangerous place. You may feel emotionally numb or indifferent to people and experiences you used to love and enjoy. You may also experience a sense of detachment from yourself or your surroundings—like an out-of-body experience or living in a dream.

Other changes are more behavioral and may include being startled easily, scanning the environment for threats, having frequent nightmares, and attempting avoidance or escape from situations that resemble the trauma, such as no longer driving because you were in a car accident, or avoiding fourth of July fireworks because they remind you of the small arms fire and incoming mortar rounds that you experienced during your combat tour. These changes tend to creep up on people over a period of several months after the traumatic event.

As you read through the experiences in the list below, check (✓) any that apply to you. As you do, be mindful that these are experiences that may follow exposure to trauma. If you don't have a history of trauma, these symptoms may not apply to you:

☐ Repetitive distressing thoughts and memories about a traumatic event

☐ Nightmares related to the event

☐ Intense and vivid flashbacks, leaving you feeling or acting as if the trauma were happening again

☐ Attempts to avoid thoughts or feelings associated with the trauma

☐ Attempts to avoid activities or external situations associated with the trauma—such as driving after you have been in a car accident

☐ An inability to experience positive emotions such as happiness, joy, love

☐ Feelings of detachment or disconnection from others (loved ones, friends)

☐ Losing interest in activities that used to give you pleasure

☐ Exaggerated negative beliefs about yourself and other people (such as "I am bad," or "People can't be trusted")

☐ Self-blame, shame, or guilt related to the trauma ("It was my fault")

☐ Always feeling on edge—difficulty falling or staying asleep, difficulty concentrating, startling easily, scanning the environment for signs of danger or threat, and irritability and outbursts of anger

☐ Elevated bodily arousal that can spiral up into a full-blown panic attack

Many people with PTSD are anxious and depressed. The trauma seems to be there as background noise all the time. Regardless of the type of trauma, people suffering from PTSD often go to great lengths to avoid thinking about the traumatic event. They also avoid any cues or situations that may remind them of the event.

Here, you may think that avoidance wouldn't be a bad thing. After all, who wants to think about some terribly awful, frightening memory from the past and, along with it, all the images and painful feelings? Unfortunately, the weight of evidence teaches us that trying to avoid thinking about the trauma, including trauma triggers around you, actually makes things worse.

The main purpose of avoidance within PTSD is to prevent reexperiencing the emotions and psychological pain associated with the trauma. The paradox, of course, is that it's next to impossible to keep painful memories from popping into our awareness, which is why avoidance isn't a lasting solution. Yet, many continue to avoid thinking about the trauma, because it offers short-term relief. Over time, avoidance grows to infect many areas of life that may have little to do with the original trauma, and ultimately ends up greatly restricting people's lives.

Sandra, a forty-three-year-old real estate broker, has struggled with PTSD since being in a horrific car accident several years ago. Her story shows how PTSD and avoidance of trauma reminders can interfere with just about all aspects of your life.

■ Sandra's Story

I was on my way to show a house to a couple who were planning to move to the area. There's a big intersection in that part of town, and I'm always careful when I drive through it. But that didn't prevent my car from being hit. The crash seemed to come out of nowhere, and as I think about it now, it feels like time slowed down—like everything was going in slow motion. Well, except for my heart rate right now—it's going through the roof! After that, all I remember is waking up hanging upside down suspended by my seat belt. I sort of recall paramedics and firefighters trying to get me out of my car. Later, the police told me that I was hit broadside by a drunk driver in a pickup truck. I ended up with a totaled car, a bunch of cuts and broken bones, and a severe concussion. I spent ten days in the hospital and haven't been the same since. I'm constantly on edge, and my sleep has been terrible with frequent nightmares of me being in a car accident and nobody coming to help me. All I see is me dying a slow painful death alone. My desire not to drive anymore has caused a lot of problems. The biggie is that I can't do my job, which has led to financial problems. It also put a lot of pressure on my husband. He picked up a second job on top of doing all the errands, including grocery shopping and driving the kids here and there. I used to help with this stuff, but now I feel I can't do it. Just the thought of driving makes me anxious and panicky. My doctor gave me some medications, but my husband said they turn me into a zombie. So I stopped taking them. The only thing that seems to help me forget is drinking white wine. But I think I'm losing control of that too. I think I won't be able to live a normal life again until I somehow get over my past.

Generalized Anxiety Disorder

Occasional worry is normal and can be useful, especially when it motivates problem solving and effective action. For instance, if you are dealing with family problems or poor health, or are struggling with lack of money and resources, worry may motivate you to come up with a plan to tackle your problems and do something about them. This is not typical of people who suffer with generalized anxiety disorder (GAD).

With GAD, worry is experienced as excessive and pervasive, often extending beyond typical concerns like family issues or health. This relentless worrying is difficult to control and channel into any effective action plan. Not surprisingly, people with GAD commonly report more worry and anxiety when feeling stressed and overwhelmed by everyday life experiences, and this worrying causes significant distress or impairs functioning across many life domains.

Approximately 9 percent of the United States population will suffer from GAD at some point in their life (Kessler et al. 2012), with females outnumbering males two to one. GAD typically develops slowly, over time, often beginning at an earlier age than other anxiety disorders. Because of this, many GAD sufferers will report that they've "always been a worrier" and "an anxious person."

As you read through the experiences in the following list, check (✓) all that apply to you:

☐ Excessive anxiety and worry about a number of events or activities

☐ Inability to stop worrying even when it's unproductive

☐ Using worry to reduce anxiety (see explanation below)

☐ Restlessness, feeling keyed up or on edge

☐ Muscle tension

☐ Being easily fatigued

☐ Difficulty concentrating

☐ Irritability or edginess

☐ Difficulties with sleep

People with GAD often have a pervasive feeling that they can do little to predict and control stressful events in their lives, including future events and outcomes, so they end up worrying about them. Many GAD sufferers also believe that worry is useful because it helps them "prepare for the worst." Some also think that worry will prevent bad things from happening or help in figuring out how to prevent bad things from happening in the future.

It used to be thought that people worry to avoid unpleasant imagery and physical tension associated with anxiety (Bandelow et al. 2013; Borkovec, Alcaine, and Behar 2004). Now, we know that there's more to worrying than simply avoidance. Worry also serves as a more general coping strategy to prepare for the possibility of things going terribly, horribly wrong. Because worrying leaves people feeling chronically distressed and anxious, there isn't much room to feel even worse should something bad actually happen (Newman and Llera 2011).

This coping strategy works in the short run—it buys the person some relief—yet in the long run, it doesn't work. People get caught in a loop of worry. They tend to experience even more intense anxiety followed by efforts to reduce anxiety by engaging in more worrying. All the while, they are unable to work through their problems and arrive at practical solutions. Samuel's case highlights this vicious cycle.

Samuel is a thirty-five-year-old IT specialist working for a state university—a job that feeds right into his lifelong struggle with worry and anxiety.

■ Samuel's Story

I went into IT thinking that the precision of technology would help me feel more secure and less anxious. Honestly, my experience has been the exact opposite of that. At work, I'm responsible for the security of our university network. I'm constantly worrying about the next hacker, virus, and phishing scam, and what would happen if they penetrated our network. I understand that some worry is part of my job. But I still worry even when we do everything right, and I spend way too much time doing my own research on the latest network threats. This has caused problems with my boss about my time management. But work is only a part of my anxiety issues. Since I was a kid, I've always been the worrier in the family. I can take the smallest thing and blow it completely out of proportion. It's like I get on what I call my worry train and can't get off and stay off. Most of the time I worry about things that are unlikely and unimportant—like the other day when I had a routine physical and some blood work. I waited a week for the lab results. During that week, I was consumed with thoughts like What if I do have some mysterious, hidden illness, and it takes me out? When I got the news that my lab work was all good, I felt a little relief, but then I still went online to double-check what all the numbers mean or could mean. All of this is just the tip of the iceberg when it comes to my anxiety. You name it, I'll find a way to worry about it. My sleep is terrible too—I lie in bed for hours because I can't shut my mind off.

ANXIETY DISORDERS HAVE MUCH IN COMMON

Each of the anxiety disorders we've covered may seem unique and different from the others. But don't let the apparent differences fool you. It turns out that the similarities are much more important than the minor variations when it comes to helping people like you. This is also true if you struggle with anxiety but haven't been given a formal diagnosis. Have a look at the list of similarities below to get a sense of what we mean:

- **Anxiety and fear are triggered by something.** There are an infinite number of possible triggers for anxiety and fear, including stress. The triggers can spring forth from within you (thoughts, images, memories, or bodily sensations), from the world around you, or from a combination of both. Some anxiety problems have clear triggers. Examples of anxiety problems with obvious triggers include specific phobias, social anxiety disorder, and PTSD. With panic disorder, OCD, and even GAD, the triggers tend to be subtler and more difficult to spot. Your anxiety and fear are triggered by something, even if you don't know what those triggers are. The triggers are there and simply need to be revealed.

- **Duration and intensity of anxiety and fear ebb and flow.** The human body is not designed to sustain anxiety and fear 24/7. In panic disorder, specific phobias, and social anxiety disorder, the fear and accompanying physical changes are intense but relatively short-lived—typically no more than half an hour and rarely beyond one hour. People who experience such difficulties may report the feelings lasting longer, but this has more to do with our minds than our bodies. Our bodies cannot keep up panic or extreme anxiety for long periods of time. In GAD, the anxiety and related physical reactions are relatively less intense, and they persist over much longer periods of time than fear. In OCD and PTSD, anxiety and tension may vary greatly in intensity and duration over time. None of it lasts forever.

- **Fear is fear, and anxiety is anxiety.** All anxiety disorders and anxiety problems include fear, anxiety, or both. You may think that fear in panic disorder is different from fear in PTSD or a phobia. Or that the experience of anxiety in GAD is fundamentally different from anxiety across other anxiety disorders. But this is not so. Fear is fear. Anxiety is anxiety. Both emotions characterize all anxiety disorders. And, at a basic level, the nature of fear and anxiety that people with anxiety disorders talk about is identical to fear and anxiety experienced from time to time by people without anxiety disorders.

- **Similar treatments work for all anxiety problems.** If anxiety problems were truly different in kind and substance, you'd expect there to be special treatments to match each unique anxiety problem. But research shows that similar treatment strategies work for all anxiety disorders. In fact, most effective treatments for anxiety problems share a small set of common exercises and skill-building tools. We've wrapped those effective elements into this book.

This list highlights what we've learned from research over the last decade or so. It shows that anxiety disorders have some striking commonalities. Yet the most important commonality didn't make it to our list. We left it out deliberately. It's time to state it boldly: nearly all people with anxiety disorders struggle to avoid feeling anxious or afraid.

Avoidant struggle turns out to be the most toxic element of all anxiety disorders. Not only does avoidance constrict lives, but it also transforms anxiety from being a normal human experience into a life-shattering problem. You got a glimpse of where avoidance can take you with the cartoons in chapter 1. We'll focus more on this critical issue in chapter 8.

OTHER PROBLEMS WITH ANXIETY DISORDERS

Studies in the United States and elsewhere around the world show that 60 percent of people with one anxiety disorder also have at least one other anxiety disorder or depression-related diagnosis, including drug abuse (Goldstein-Piekarski, Williams, and Humphreys 2016). Quite a few are also taking some form of medication for anxiety or depression. We cover these concerns below because there's a good chance that some might apply to you.

Depression

Depression is a persistent mood state where people feel very sad, "down and empty," worthless, and hopeless about the future. Some people say that depression feels like a black curtain of despair has come down over their lives; just about everything they do is cast in darkness by this curtain. Many question whether their life situation will ever improve.

Lack of energy and fatigue are common complaints, and many report difficulties concentrating, remembering, and making decisions. Many also have sleep difficulties. Others feel irritable and restless all the time for no apparent reason. They often lose interest in hobbies and activities that they once enjoyed, including sex.

Depression is by far the most common co-occurring emotional problem experienced by people with anxiety disorders. In fact, about 81 percent of people with an anxiety disorder will also experience significant depression at some point (ter Meulen et al. 2021). At times depression may develop before an anxiety disorder, but it's more common for depression to creep up on people after they've been dealing with an anxiety disorder for a while.

Given the way anxiety and fear can get in the way of meaningful life activities, it's not surprising that people start to think and feel that life is no longer enjoyable or worth living. The good news is that this workbook can help lift the veil depression may have on you. Our own research, which we discussed in the prologue, looked at people with severe anxiety and severe depression. You may recall that many showed significant improvements in their depression when they worked with this book.

Alcohol

Virtually all people with anxiety problems engage in similar strategies to cope with their anxiety—strategies that have not worked very well and have caused more problems in the long run. For instance, men tend to self-medicate their anxiety problem with alcohol, often with the hope that it'll make their life situation more bearable (Barlow 2004). But women also use alcohol to cope with anxiety. This self-defeating strategy is chosen by at least one in every five people with an anxiety disorder.

As with avoidance, this tactic blunts emotional and psychological distress for a short while, but over time the distress comes right back (often worse than before), and now the person has two problems—a more entrenched anxiety disorder and budding alcoholism.

If you think that your drinking is in the service of managing your anxiety, fear, and even stress, we strongly encourage you to take stock and seek additional help if necessary. As you work on learning the skills in this book, you may find that drinking to take the edge off no longer has a purpose. You may also find that you're unable to stop drinking alcohol, even after using this workbook, because you've developed a dependence on alcohol. Take this as another sign to get the support and help you need.

Medical Conditions

Many medical conditions can mimic signs and sensations associated with anxiety and fear. For this reason, it's best to consult with a trained professional to rule out any medical conditions or possible drug-related factors that may be contributing to your anxiety and related concerns.

Examples of medical disorders that can trigger symptoms of panic or anxiety include thyroid problems, balance disorders, seizure disorders, asthma, and other respiratory or heart conditions. Use of stimulants (like cocaine, caffeine, diet pills, and certain other medications) and other drugs (like marijuana), along with withdrawal from alcohol and other drugs, can also trigger panic-like feelings.

So before assuming that you have an anxiety disorder, talk with your doctor. Get a full medical workup to help determine whether there's a physical cause for your problems. You can also think of this as a good way to take care of yourself. Once physical causes are ruled out, you can be much more confident about using the strategies described in this book.

Medications

Many people with anxiety disorders are prescribed medication. You may be one of them. Even if you were never diagnosed, your doctor may have given you medication for your anxiety symptoms. In fact, we know from our research that about 40 percent of readers were taking prescription medication for their anxiety and/or depression while using this workbook. So, if this applies to you, you have nothing to worry about.

We also know from our research and that of others that medications can be helpful, but they're not curative. It may also surprise you to learn that researchers are now questioning the very idea that anxiety and depression are caused by a chemical imbalance in the brain and that medications somehow correct that imbalance.

What we do know is that medications can offer some people short-term symptom relief. Studies also show that people tend to do worse in the long run when on medications alone or in combination with gold-standard treatments like CBT. In fact, the best long-term outcomes are found in people who work to make significant changes on their own, with or without the help of a therapist, using proven strategies.

This is also not the time for you to stop taking your medication as prescribed. You should first consult with your doctor before making any changes to your medications. The good news is that you can benefit from this workbook even if you're taking medications for anxiety, depression, or both.

As you work with this workbook, you may want to reflect on why you're taking antianxiety or antidepressant medication. Look at your intentions here. Are you taking medication to get rid of or to control your anxiety? Look also at how the medication is working. Are you anxiety- and depression-free while taking your medication?

Many people struggling with anxiety and depression do not wish to be taking medications their entire lives. You may feel that way too. Some of the skills in this workbook will help you learn to be with your anxiety and depression just as they are. This new way of relating with your emotional life may then lead you to have a conversation with your doctor about reducing or discontinuing your medication entirely.

WHAT'S YOUR PROBLEM WITH ANXIETY?

To get unstuck from your current situation, you don't need to have been diagnosed with an anxiety disorder. Instead, it's much more important for you to identify what is feeding your anxiety and keeping you stuck.

The key is to start with the most problematic aspects of your anxiety. To help you along, ask yourself this question: *What are the most disturbing and interfering aspects of my problem with anxiety?* Find your answer to this question by going over the checklists in this chapter. Then, write down what stands out to you in the space below.

Consider symptoms and behaviors that lead you to pull out of your life in a flash, where you'll try like crazy to avoid experiencing anxiety or fear. You can also go back and review the case examples to help you choose events, situations, and behaviors to work with later on.

_____

_____

_____

_____

_____

_____

_____

LIFE-ENHANCEMENT EXERCISES

For this week, we invite you to do the following:

- Do one of the centering exercises daily. Simply choose the one you like best.

- Spend time with the material in this chapter.

- Before moving on, be as clear as you can about symptoms and behaviors that you struggle with most and how they've made your life challenging.

THE TAKE-HOME MESSAGE

Fear and anxiety are two unpleasant emotions that can be healthy and adaptive. Both emotions propel us into action and serve the purpose of keeping us alive and out of trouble. Labeling yourself with a diagnosis for your anxiety problem will not help you or make your life more livable. Diagnostic labels are just that, words, and these words can often be self-limiting. So, instead of playing the label game, we're going to help you identify the root of the most problematic aspects of your anxiety problem. For instance, what is it that turns your fear, anxiety, worry, or obsession into the life-restricting problem it has become? What is it that you have been struggling with? Facing these questions squarely is the key to making changes that will help you get your life back.

Discovering the Root of My Anxiety Problem(s)

Reflections:

- Receiving a professional diagnosis won't help me get my life back.

- What I need to do is look into how the drama of managing and avoiding anxiety plays out in my life, so I can start taking steps to do something about that.

Inquiries:

- What exactly are my problems with anxiety?

- What are the most disturbing and interfering aspects of my problem with anxiety?

CHAPTER 3

Letting Go of the Myths About Anxiety

Think about any attachments that are depleting your emotional reserves.
Consider letting them go.

—Oprah Winfrey

It seems like every day we're learning something new about anxiety and its disorders. This entire workbook stands on the shoulders of hundreds, if not thousands, of research studies. Each has explored what turns anxiety and fear into life-shattering problems and, more importantly, what you can do about it.

You probably also know quite a bit about anxiety already. Some of this you know from your lived experience. You may have picked up other pearls of wisdom from newspaper and magazine articles, books, TV, the internet, social media, conversations with family members and others, or from what your doctor has told you.

Along the way, it's likely that you've come across the idea that anxiety disorders are a disease, just like diabetes or cancer, or that some people inherit anxiety disorders. You may have heard that anxiety disorders can be treated with herbal remedies or by changing your diet. Others have told you that anxiety disorders are caused by your brain's neurochemicals run amok, so you need medications to repair chemical imbalances within your faulty brain.

In fact, you may feel overwhelmed by all the new research and sound bites about the causes and potential cures for anxiety. Scientists and the media are equally guilty of promoting unhelpful messages. Sadly, there's no solid evidence that magnets, aromatherapy, Bach flower therapy, biofeedback gadgets, brain wave synchronizers, thought field therapy, hypnosis, homeopathy, passionflower tea, or special diets cure anxiety and panic. In fact, even our best available, scientifically supported treatments do not cure anxiety in the sense of making it go away and for good. So, when you see a claim of a new cure, please be mindful of your wallet.

Many of these claims imply that experiencing intense fear and anxiety is abnormal. You might even believe this yourself. It's easy to think that such feelings make you weak, broken, or put you on the verge of losing it and going crazy.

Westernized cultures also promote the idea that you can and should learn to manage and control your anxious thoughts and feelings if you want to be happy and thrive. Again, this message implies that anxiety isn't okay, and that because you're feeling it you're not okay too.

These are all common beliefs about anxiety, and even some mental health professionals accept them. Yet none of them are true. Each is a myth or, at best, a partial truth. They're unhelpful because they keep you and others like you stuck in old patterns that don't work. They leave you wanting, waiting, and struggling to get a foothold. They feed patterns of thinking that you're unlike most people who seemingly glide through life happy and carefree. This isn't so.

FOUR COMMON MYTHS ABOUT ANXIETY

Let's take a look at the myths and reveal them for what they are.

Myth #1: Anxiety Problems Are Biological and Hereditary

Too often we hear people say, "Anxiety runs in my family, so that's why I'm anxious." Or, "My doctor said my anxiety disorder is caused by my family's genes, so the best I can do is take medication to manage it." You may even think this way yourself. You shouldn't fault yourself for that, because all of us are bombarded by such messages, particularly in the popular media. They sound credible, especially when you hear them from "experts" or medical professionals. Fortunately, both claims also turn out to be false.

Yes, it is true that anxiety often runs in families, but that's largely because of learned behavior, not because of genes. You may inherit some predisposition to be anxious or afraid, just like you inherit predispositions to be outgoing, introverted, intelligent, muscular, or athletic. But inheriting a *predisposition* to be anxious is not the same thing as inheriting an anxiety *disorder*.

In fact, there's no compelling evidence that you or anyone else is born with any anxiety disorder. At best, genes contribute about 30 to 40 percent to your anxiety problems (Leonardo and Hen 2006). What this also means is that about 60 to 70 percent of your difficulties have little to do with your biology or genes. In fact, newer work with epigenetics is showing that genetics are not as fixed as we once thought. Many genes seem to operate like light switches, turning on and off in response to the environment and what we do. This work teaches us that your genes are not your destiny. Whatever your genetic makeup, there is room to grow and change.

Even the idea that anxiety and depression are caused by chemical imbalances and that medications correct those imbalances has been challenged and refuted. We also once thought that the chemical imbalance theory was an established scientific fact, until we learned that it's really a metaphor to justify the sale of medications for various human woes. We share this with you now because so many people think that they have a faulty brain that requires medication. We're here to tell you that the weight of current scientific thinking says this too is a myth.

The bulk of what makes anxiety a psychiatric problem has nothing to do with your biology or genetics. That other 60 to 70 percent has to do with how you relate with your anxiety and fear—what you do about your anxious thoughts and feelings. This is the more important part, because it's something you can control and change. You cannot change your genes, nor can you change your biology in any permanent sense with a pill. But you can change your life (and with that also your biology) by changing what you do. This is why we'll focus on helping you work on what you can control and change—your actions—what you do when you have anxious feelings.

Myth #2: Intense Anxiety Is Abnormal

People often seek help for anxiety because they don't like how they think or feel. The anxiety and fear seem overwhelming, the painful memories too much to bear, the thoughts and worries paralyzing or next to impossible to turn off. In a word, anxiety is too intense.

> People don't inherit anxiety disorders.

It's certainly true that intense anxiety tends to go hand in hand with all anxiety disorders. It's also true that intense anxiety doesn't constitute an anxiety disorder. We need the capacity to feel intense emotions like anxiety and fear. All humans are wired to experience a range of emotions at varying levels of intensity. It would be abnormal if this weren't so.

As you saw in chapter 2, intense fear has one purpose—to ready you for action when faced with real danger or risk of harm. Life-threatening events such as combat, sexual assault, abuse, accidents, and natural disasters fall into this category. In these situations, most people will experience intense fear. Even strongly felt anxiety may help you prepare now for future challenges. Without the capacity to feel such emotions intensely, we wouldn't have survived as a species. These reactions are 100 percent normal.

Many people experience intense anxiety, even panic attacks, in their daily lives *and* continue to do what's important to them. Intensely felt emotions need not be a barrier to the life you want to lead. They can be welcomed in as a necessary *part* of you. This is why we're going to help you learn new ways of relating with your anxious thoughts and feelings and how to take them with you. If you're willing, this approach will get you unstuck and moving toward the life you want. Going forward, keep reminding yourself that intense anxiety doesn't make anxiety a problem. Same with fear.

Myth #3: Anxiety Is a Sign of Weakness

Anxiety isn't a sign of weakness, personality defect, poor character, laziness, or lack of motivation. Anyone can get stuck and offtrack because of emotional or psychological pain. The experience of pain is built into the human condition.

You may buy into the idea that anxiety is a sign of weakness because other people seem so well put together. You see others making it, doing things that you'd like to do, seemingly without the shadow of anxiety hanging over their heads. This great illusion is fueled by two sources. The first has to do with the tendency for our minds to jump to conclusions based on very limited information. When you see and interact with others, you may not see them as anxious or actively suffering. You may think, *Why can't I be that way?* And next, *Something must be wrong with me.*

What is needed here is some perspective. Imagine that you're able to shadow one person who you think has it all together. You can watch this person's every move 24/7 and know what they're thinking and feeling at any time. If you were able to do this, you'd find out that this person is not so different from you.

Anxiety isn't a sign of weakness.

As you get to know this person's humanity, you'd see someone who experiences a whole range of thoughts and feelings, just like you—pleasant, unpleasant, and everything in between. You'd also notice that this person needs to eat, drink, sleep, and use the bathroom, just like you. They, like you, will at times feel frustrated, be worried about this or that, or experience sadness, loneliness, regret, and anger. At times, you'd see that they, too, also feel anxious or afraid.

The second source that fuels the weakness myth is social comparison. When you narrowly view your life as full of anxiety and emotional pain and see others as dancing through the lily fields of life, seemingly happy and carefree, you'll naturally feel that something is wrong with you. You'll think that you're missing something they have.

The truth is that you have everything you need. You aren't broken. The capacity for change lies within you. You and only you are responsible for what you do with your precious time and energy. This is why we'll be nurturing your capacity for responsibility. With that, you'll create change in your life by refocusing your time, energy, and resources on what you can control and change in your life—the things you do with your hands, feet, and mouth.

Myth #4: Anxiety Must Be Managed to Live a Vital Life

Of all the myths, this one is the most damaging. It's fueled by social rules and expectations, or what we call the *culture of feel-goodism*. These rules set up emotional and physical pain as barriers to a life lived well. They also encourage us to struggle. The message goes something like this:

1. It's normal to be happy and thriving in life.

2. Discomfort—physical, emotional, psychological—isn't normal.

3. In fact, discomfort is a barrier to happiness and life fulfillment.

4. So, if you're feeling any discomfort, then you need to do something about it to be happy and thrive.

5. And once you are thinking and feeling better, then your life will improve for the better.

6. But, if you're unable to get a handle on your discomfort, you'll never be happy.

This is a trap.

The bait for the trap is the emotional and psychological discomfort you experience with anxiety, panic, worries, and unwanted thoughts or memories. Because of your cultural conditioning, your mind probably tells you that your discomfort isn't just discomfort. It's *bad* discomfort. It's a problem.

Your mind not only judges discomfort as unacceptable but also links it with not being able to do what you care about. This is your cultural conditioning again. So, when anxiety discomfort shows up, you go after it to weaken it or drive it away. You also try to prevent *bad* discomfort from showing up in the future, because you've learned that this is necessary to live the kind of life you want. In truth, this is a big lie.

EXERCISE: Don't Think About a Pink Elephant

This brief exercise will help you see what trying to suppress and control unwanted thoughts gets you. Go ahead and get in a comfortable position. Now, when you're ready, we'd like you to close your eyes and try not to think about a PINK ELEPHANT! Try hard. Give yourself a few minutes to really work at it. After you've given it a go, open your eyes and read on.

You're not alone if you found this task difficult or impossible. That's because you cannot do what the instruction says without thinking of the thing you're not supposed to think about. Put another way, the thought **Don't think about a PINK ELEPHANT** is itself a thought about pink elephants. So, there you are, stuck with the very thing you don't want to think about.

Your mind may have come up with other clever tactics to accomplish the goal of not thinking about a pink elephant. Maybe you tried thinking about something else. This seems reasonable. Yet how did your mind do that? How did you know that the other thought was not a pink elephant? In order to think of something that's clearly not a pink elephant, your brain needs to make a comparison. For instance, a bear is not a pink elephant. So, there you are again, thinking about pink elephants and now bears too.

Your mental programming has lots of links that surface automatically, just as the thoughts of pink elephants did, because you've learned them. Here are a few. Go ahead and fill in the blanks without giving it much thought.

Twinkle, twinkle, little _____   Practice makes _____

Don't spill the _____   Actions speak louder than _____

Look before you _____   The early bird gets the _____

Now, we'd like you to pick one of these statements and read it slowly, but don't think about the word that completes the phrase. For instance, read "Twinkle, twinkle, little" but don't think _____ the next word. What happened? Could you do it? Let's take this a step further.

Imagine that "star" is one of those really distressing thoughts, bodily sensations, feelings, or memories that you struggle with and wish not to have. You're now in a situation where your automatic programming kicks in. Here it comes—"Twinkle, twinkle, little _____ "—but you can't have what comes next. What do you suppose will happen here? You end up with more of the thing you don't want to experience. You may also try to avoid it in the future.

When you take the bait, what happens to the discomfort and your life? You are devoting enormous time, energy, and resources to keeping the anxiety and panic at bay. You keep doing this because it has often bought you some temporary relief. You also do it because this is what you've been taught to do in our culture, even if it doesn't work as a long-term solution.

Anxiety management and avoidance leave you feeling safe and less anxious in the short term and greatly limit what you can do. This inaction is a problem.

If you suffer from panic disorder, then you may know what this is like. Having a panic attack at the grocery store or elsewhere is a highly unpleasant experience. And it may lead you to do things to prevent it from happening again: stop shopping, shop with a "safe" person and never alone, only go to the store late in the evening when few people are around in case you panic again, and so on. During all of this, you may be concentrating on relaxing, as you also watch for signs of a possible panic attack.

If your difficulties are with social anxiety, you may take many steps to minimize or avoid having anxiety in social encounters. This is hard to do in a highly social world like ours and so can be quite crippling. Imagine going about your day without interacting with people for fear that you might panic or humiliate or embarrass yourself. Now imagine how going about your day might feel knowing the truth that none of us can control how other people respond to us.

Time spent trying to manage and control anxiety is time and energy away from doing things that you care deeply about. So anxiety management and control actually double your discomfort: on top of the discomfort of more anxiety, you also get the pain of loss or regret that comes from an unfulfilled life. This other discomfort will creep up on you over time when you take a pass on doing something that's important to you because of fear and anxiety. Both forms of discomfort are a natural consequence of fighting a battle with your unpleasant thoughts and feelings.

But don't fault yourself for doing this. Everyone can get stuck trying to make their discomfort go away. The culture of feel-goodism is pernicious. And many studies show that people get more of the very thing they don't want when they try to push it out of their mind.

So, when you don't want anxious thoughts and feelings, you'll get more of them. And the more you don't want them, the more you're stuck with them. We'll elaborate on how this works in a moment. For now, the important thing to remember is that these actions fuel your anxiety and slam the trapdoor shut on your life.

WHERE THE MYTHS WILL TAKE YOU IF YOU LET THEM

The myths are, in a sense, like a sticky spider web. When you get caught up in the web, the natural reaction is to struggle to get out. But that just leaves you more tangled and stuck in anxiety and cut off from the life that you want to lead.

Here, it's important to start learning to trust your lived experience and not what your mind tells you to do. Take a moment to reflect on your lived experience. Have any of your tried-and-true coping strategies worked in the long run? Does your experience tell you that they'll work if you just work harder, longer, or better? Do you want to be about dealing with anxiety for the rest of your life? Haven't you worked and suffered long enough?

■ Sharon's Story

Sharon's story illustrates where the myths can take you if you let them. She came to us at the age of forty-five after twenty years of crippling struggle with anxiety, panic, and depression. She believed that something was biologically wrong with her. She thought of herself as the kind of person who had been dealt a bad hand—a life filled with too much emotional pain and anguish. Her runaway mind was constantly feeding her doom and gloom, self-blame, and negativity. Sharon didn't think she had much of a chance for a bright future. She saw her life ticking by and feared being put in a hospital, medicated, doped up, and cut off from her children and her life.

Still, Sharon had not given up. She had been on and off antidepressant and antianxiety medication and in and out of cognitive behavioral therapy, often finding that treatment left her with a renewed sense of hope, a brief sojourn from the crippling panic, wrenching anxiety, agoraphobia, and disturbing thoughts. She had bought a sun lamp to stave off the depression. She had invested hundreds of dollars in professional and self-help books about anxiety disorders, belonged to many online support groups, and even attended seminars.

For about two years, Sharon had been living better and seemed to feel better too. Armed with a solid set of tools to keep her anxiety and fear at bay, she was able to readily challenge her negative thoughts, relax away the tension, dismiss the worry, and breathe herself out of panic. And she had the sun lamp and the books to read when she found herself in an emotional pinch. These strategies seemed to work, but she never fully escaped the lurking sense that someday, somewhere, the strategies wouldn't work anymore—and then the shadow of anxiety and depression would return and take over. And that's exactly what happened and what ultimately led Sharon to us.

Sharon was at a tipping point, and she knew it. For the first time in her life, she was ready to look for new answers instead of old solutions. This shift began when Sharon finally asked herself this question: Can I learn to live with feelings and thoughts that I dislike and not allow them to control me and what I do?

LETTING GO OF THE MYTHS

Recently, while packing for a family vacation to the beach, Sharon stuffed a duffle bag full of her old safety myths: vitamins for her anxiety, her iPhone loaded with relaxation tracks and self-help lectures, earplugs to blot out the noise of her kids playing in the hotel room, a sun lamp to ward off depression, and a dozen or so books on anxiety and its disorders. The weight of her baggage was enormous, literally and emotionally.

It turned out that all this antianxiety gear was unnecessary. Over the weekend, Sharon didn't open her duffle bag once. With a chuckle, she said, "I certainly had times when I felt anxious and had anxious thoughts. And then I reminded myself that I didn't want to be about what was in the duffle bag."

For Sharon, packing her duffle bag was about buying into the myth that she must control her anxiety to enjoy her trip and live her life. Letting go of that myth allowed her to spend her time outside, playing with her husband and children on the beach, going for sunset walks, and reading a fun book. She went out to dinner and took the kids to a Sunday matinee. She even had a chance to share quiet conversation with her husband over a glass of wine on the balcony of her hotel room.

At times she felt good while doing all these things she cared deeply about. And at other times she was quite anxious about the possibility of having a panic attack. Importantly, she was unwilling to spend time struggling with anxiety, panic, and the negative news that her mind fed her from time to time. She gave herself some space to have all those experiences without trying to change them. Her weekend left her feeling alive!

Sharon's story is typical in many ways. Your particular story may be different. But if you also believe that your life has shrunk to the size of a postage stamp, then you may be just as stuck as Sharon was. Is it possible that, like Sharon, you don't need to think and feel better first in order to live better? Are you willing to let go of the myths you hold on to about anxiety?

Sharon found her answers not by blindly trusting what we said. In fact, she had serious doubts about what our treatment program could offer her. The ideas were new, a bit strange, and challenged what she believed could and ought to be done about her anxiety and her life.

We didn't ask Sharon to stop worrying or resolve her doubts. And we won't ask you to do that either. All we ask is that you soften to the possibility that your old ideas about the solutions to your anxiety problems may be doing you more harm than good.

As Sharon began doing the exercises in this book, she learned that things could be different when she approached her anxiety and her life in a new way and with different priorities. You have this option too.

WHAT FUELS THE MYTHS AND KEEPS THEM ALIVE?

There are four key factors that fuel the myths about anxiety, turn anxiety into a problem, and keep you stuck.

The Fusion Mind Trap

Like every human being, you have the capacity to become fused or tangled up with your thoughts. When you fuse with your thoughts, you'll tend to treat them as if they were the same thing as the experiences or events they describe.

For instance, the word "panic" may conjure up all sorts of associations. These may include images of having a heart attack, death, fainting, going crazy, losing it, or being carted off to a psychiatric hospital. Your mind will also throw judgment and evaluation into these associations, such as panic is bad, dangerous, weak, stupid, humiliating, and so on. Each of these words have their own associations too, many of them quite negative.

What's important to see here is that the word "panic" is not a real panic attack, nor is it the same as the associations and evaluations linked with the word. The word "panic" is just a word. The evaluation "bad" is just an evaluation. You could choose to treat them as such. Or you could respond to the word, its associations, and evaluations as if they are more than that.

When you go beyond seeing words as words, you're buying into the illusion your mind creates. The thoughts shift from being thoughts to being something dangerously serious. And when that happens, you'll often find yourself trapped in old behavior patterns that are neither helpful nor in your best interest. We call this a *mind trap*.

Think of fusion as buying into the literal meaning of thoughts when they're unhelpful, leading you to do things that are far from what you want to be doing or really care about. You can also fuse with emotions, urges, and physical sensations. Don't worry if you're having a hard time wrapping your head around what fusion is. We'll come back to this concept and how to defuse from unhelpful thoughts more experientially throughout the book.

Fusion is important to know about, because anxious suffering is often set into motion when you feed your unpleasant thoughts and feelings by getting tangled up with them. When you allow your mind to take you down the fusion road unchecked, you will naturally react strongly to what your mind feeds you, and give thoughts more importance than they deserve. This can keep you stuck.

EXERCISE: Getting Tangled Up with Anxiety

To get a sense of this process, take a moment to complete the following exercise. Select a thought, worry, emotional experience, or memory that's particularly upsetting for you. Once you have that in mind, jot down events or experiences that tend to go along with it. Here's how Mark, who suffers from strong anxiety and panic attacks, did this exercise.

Mark's Experience	What Comes to Mind
Panic/strong anxiety	1. Chest tightness, can't catch my breath
	2. Focus on getting out of where I am
	3. Heart is pounding, super sweaty
	4. Can't be in a crowd, drive a car, go near heights
	5. Think I might be going crazy

As Mark reflected on his past experience with panic, he noticed that he would often buy into his anxious thoughts and feelings and then try to eliminate them. When he did that, he also got everything else on his list and then some. He felt more anxious. (Remember the pink elephant.) Worse, he became the very thing he wished not to be by fusing his sense of being with his anxiety, as in "I'm anxious."

In fact, Mark told us, "I'm an anxious wreck." In feeding that thought, he had become a person who was not only anxious but also incapable of being in a crowd, driving a car, and going to work. He had also begun to think of himself as disabled. No surprise, given that he had fused with the very things he most disliked, including the word "disabled."

Now it's your turn to examine your experience.

My Experience	What Comes to Mind
	1.
	2.
	3.
	4.
	5.

If you're anything like Mark, you probably assign significant weight to anxiety-provoking thoughts or feelings. That's because you've learned to buy into what your mind tells you about your experience. The more you do that, the more you become fused with the label and evaluations and trapped by your mind.

You might be thinking, *Are they telling me that my fear and anxiety aren't real?* Absolutely not. The bodily sensations, the thoughts, and the images are all real, in the sense of being genuine aspects of your experience.

What we're asking is for you to look closely at what you're responding to. Are you responding to the images as images, thoughts as thoughts, sensations as sensations, and memories as memories, *as they are,* unedited and untainted by negative evaluations?

Or are your actions steered by judgments and evaluations of these experiences—the stuff your mind feeds you about them? We'd also like you to consider whether you must respond to experiences as though they're what your mind says they are (the racing heart is a heart attack and not simply a fast heartbeat), or can you treat them as actual sensations, as thoughts consisting of words, or as fleeting memories of the past?

You may have had times when you've said to yourself, *I'm weak, I'm depressed, I'm a loser,* or *I'm going crazy.* Each of these statements may seem like they describe who you are. But is that so? Are you the words your mind creates about you?

Take a moment to imagine what would happen if all of a sudden you had the thought, *I am a banana*. To find out, close your eyes for ten seconds and keep thinking the thought *I am a banana*. What happened? Perhaps you saw a yellow curved object in your mind. You may have imagined the taste of a banana. Did having that thought turn you into a banana? Is that thought any more true or false than any other thought your mind might throw at you now and then?

Intuitively, you know that your thoughts are different than the events they describe. As we teach you how to step back and defuse or disentangle a bit, you'll see that, in essence, thoughts are simply thoughts, sensations are sensations, memories are memories, and feelings are feelings—nothing more, nothing less. We'll teach you skills so that you don't "become" them.

If you feel a bit confused, be patient and skeptical about what your mind may be telling you now, and keep reading to discover for yourself what this might mean and how it can help you.

Evaluating Your Experiences

Just about everything human beings experience and do is tagged with some sort of evaluation or judgment: good versus bad, right versus wrong, happy versus sad. Media and marketing are built around helping you experience a positive evaluation of products so you will buy them. Similarly, models of health and wellness are built around the idea that emotional and psychological pain are not simply pain but "bad" pain. You can apply this habit of evaluation as readily to yourself and your private experiences as you can to most events in your world.

There's nothing wrong with evaluating your experience. We all do it. The trick is to recognize that your verbal evaluation of reality is not reality itself. To put it another way, you might call a duckling "ugly" or "cute," but that doesn't change the fact that the duckling is a duckling. This is an important point that we'll revisit throughout this book.

When you buy into and feed your negative evaluations unnecessarily, you'll often fuel your suffering unnecessarily. It just plain hurts when we evaluate ourselves and our experiences negatively—as ugly, broken, screwed up, weak, worthless, stupid, crazy, foolish, and the like.

You may not be able to control the stream of evaluations, but you can choose to feed them or not. When you make choices, always keep in mind that what you pay attention to in your life will grow and become stronger. Always put your attention on those aspects of your life that you want to grow and become stronger.

Feeding a Painful Wolf or a Compassionate Heart

Here's a short story to give you a sense of what we mean.

> *A Native American grandfather was talking to his grandson about how he felt. He said, "I feel as if I have two wolves fighting for my heart. One wolf is vengeful, angry, and violent. The*

other wolf is loving, compassionate, kind, and hopeful." The grandson asked him, "Which wolf will win the fight for your heart?" The grandfather answered, "The one I feed."

In chapter 2, we talked about anxiety and fear as being a loose collection of bodily sensations, thoughts, and behavioral predispositions, all of which tend to hang together with other events and situations you've experienced. Go back and review what you wrote down about these areas as they apply to your experience with anxiety and fear.

With these thoughts, bodily sensations, feelings, and behaviors in mind, take a moment to write down words that best describe your evaluation of them. You may think of these as bad, unwanted, unpleasant, nasty, aversive, painful, screwed up, awful, annoying, or wrenching, or you may have other words that you routinely apply to them. Don't overthink this. Just write down any judgments that immediately show up.

> *Don't feed the anxiety wolf; feed your values instead.*

Take a moment to pause and reflect. Look at what you tend to respond to more: your experiences just as they are—unedited—or your judgments and negative labels about those experiences? It will tend to be one or the other, not both. What is it for you?

When you buy into the negative evaluations, you're left with only one sensible option—to do what you can to rid yourself of the "bad" and potentially "harmful" experience. You feed your anxious wolf. Buying into judgmental labels also leads to inevitable actions. Suppose one of your judgmental thoughts was *My panic attacks are so bad, they're eventually going to kill me.* If you completely believe this thought and only react to what it seems to say, then you're left with few options. The thought says that your life is in the balance. So, you *must* do something about it. Perhaps you won't leave the house, or you'll take an antianxiety pill every few hours. The same principles are at work with obsessional thoughts that you think will come true if you don't do something about them, like *I may have come in contact with germs* or *I might harm my children.*

The bottom line is this: nothing else makes sense except to prevent what the thought suggests. But here's the rub: as soon as you do that, you'll find yourself caught in the fusion mind trap, feeding the hungry anxiety wolf one more time.

Avoiding Your Experiences

Avoiding or escaping from experiences that bring on the "bad" thoughts and feelings may leave you with a brief honeymoon from the pain and its source. In fact, this is exactly what keeps avoidance and escape behavior going. You feel better after you avoid or leave a situation, so you're more likely to do it again. The relief also tends to be fleeting. Countless studies have shown that this temporary relief makes it more likely that you'll use the same strategy the next time the "bad" anxiety or fear rears its "ugly" head.

Avoidance would make sense if the situations could actually harm or kill you. But that's not what we're talking about here. Avoidance across the anxiety disorders is about not having unpleasant psychological and emotional experiences. Such avoidance is both unnecessary and enormously costly.

For now, we'd like you to consider the possibility that the discomfort that lies beneath your "bad" anxiety and fear may not be so bad after all. In fact, it may serve a useful purpose and be a type of "growing pain." You may need it to get you moving toward the life that you so desperately want.

Reason-Giving for Your Behavior

Many people we've helped with anxiety harbor deeply rooted reasons for why they cannot do this or that. Here are a couple of examples:

- "I can't fly in a plane, because I might panic."

- "I can't be in crowds, because it's too unsafe."

The content will differ across the reasons, but all have a familiar ring to them. Each includes an "I can't" and a "because." The part right after "I can't" points to an important life experience, and the part after "because" points to the problem that seems to be getting in the way.

By now, you've probably come up with several plausible reasons why you *can't do* this or that *because* of your worries, anxieties, and fears (WAFs). These WAFs are barking at you much like a dog might do: WAF…WAF…WAF! And when others ask you why you can't do this or that, you may respond with lots of reasons that take this form—because of "WAF…WAF…WAF!"

With your WAFs in mind, we'd like you to recall what you wrote down in the introduction:

I have missed out on or am unable to _____

_____because of my anxious thoughts and feelings.

If we were to ask you, "Why can't you do that one important thing in your life?" you might respond, "Because I might panic or get too anxious, faint, lose control, get hurt, humiliate myself, break down, or act on my disturbing thoughts." WAF, WAF, WAF!

In fact, it's common for people struggling with anxiety disorders to give themself or others reasons that point to anxious thoughts and feelings. And many people will go along with what you say to be sympathetic, kind, and supportive. This only solidifies the link between your WAFs and your inability to take action.

Look what happens when you start to believe your reasons—your own stories. Like a big, fierce-looking dog, your WAFs have now turned into a barrier that stands in the way of going forward in your life. For example, if you can't fly because you might have a panic attack, the only way you'll ever fly is if you can make sure you never panic—WAF! Reasons linked with anxiety and fear now become the causes of you being stuck. And when you buy into this story line, which is easy to do in our culture, you'll be left thinking that the only way to go forward is to take care of the causes: *I must do something about my WAFs.*

We've already given you a taste of what happens when you buy into thoughts like *Don't be anxious!* In the chapters to come we'll help you get a better sense of what the struggle to control anxiety and fear has cost you. For now, let's look at some skills that will help you move with your anxiety and fear and live your life.

LEARNING TO OBSERVE YOUR EXPERIENCE

One of the most courageous things you can do when your WAFs show up is to sit still with them and not do what they tell you to do. It's courageous because the impulse to cut and run is automatic and strong. Doing nothing about them is the more difficult path. It's important to learn this skill because the urge to do something about your WAFs greatly diminishes your life. Practicing *mind watching* will teach you to become an observer of your mind rather than taking and swallowing whatever nasty-looking stuff your mind offers you.

Mind Watching

We know that observing your mind filled with WAFs isn't easy. Your mind will be screaming at you to respond as you've done in the past. Through persistent practice, however, it will get easier over time to observe and take note of thoughts, images, and urges rather than do as they say. Here's how you get started.

EXERCISE: Mind Watching

Get in a comfortable place where you won't be disturbed for about five to ten minutes. Begin by closing your eyes and taking a few slow, deep breaths. Keep this up throughout the entire exercise. Imagine your mind is a medium-sized white room with two doors. Thoughts come in through the front door and leave out the back door. First, watch each thought as it enters. Keep on watching to see what it's doing next. Don't do anything with it.

Your only task here is simply to watch thoughts as they enter. Don't analyze them. Don't engage or argue with them, and don't believe or disbelieve them either. Just acknowledge having each thought—that's all. Acknowledge *and* do nothing but watch. Thoughts can be a fleeting moment in your mind, a brief visitor in the white room. Keep on watching each thought until it leaves. When it wants to go, let it go and don't try to hold on to it.

If you find that you're judging yourself for having a particular thought, then just notice that. Don't argue with your mind's judgment. Just notice it for what it is, and label it: *Thinking— there's thinking*. The key to this exercise is to notice judgmental and other unwanted thoughts rather than getting caught up in them. You'll know if you're getting caught up in them by your emotional reactions and by how long each thought stays in the room.

Keep breathing...and keep watching. A thought is just a thought. A thought doesn't require you to react. It doesn't make you do anything. It doesn't mean you're less of a person for having it. Again, watch and notice your thoughts and treat them as if they were visitors passing in and out of the white room. Let them have their brief moment on the stage. They're fine the way they are—including the judging thoughts and any other uninvited visitors. The important thing is to let them leave when they're ready to go and then greet and label the next thought... and the next.

Continue this exercise until you sense some emotional distance from your thoughts. Wait until even the judgments are just a moment in the room—no longer important, no longer requiring action. Practice this exercise at least once a day.

Take Your Mind and Body for a Walk

Another way to learn to be a skillful observer of your thoughts and feelings is to practice moving *with* them instead of *because of* them. To practice doing that, think of taking your mind and body for a walk. Start your practice by literally going outside for a walk, for fifteen minutes or longer, without listening to music.

EXERCISE: Mindful Walking

As you walk, you'll notice that you don't need to think much about what your legs and body are doing. They move with you more or less automatically. Here, we're going to learn to bring mindful awareness to this experience.

As you begin this activity, focus on your breathing—deeply in and out—as you did with some of the centering exercises we covered earlier. Walk naturally and bring awareness to the rhythm of your steps and how your body feels as it moves. If your mind wanders to other things, just notice that. Then, gently bring your attention back to the experience of walking.

Notice the feel of your feet as they meet the ground with each step. Move your awareness to your hip area—experience how your hips move with each stride. What sensations are there? Then move further up to your midsection, and allow yourself to feel all the movements there too. See how your body is in perfect rhythm and flow.

Notice how you're moving with your thoughts and feelings too—all of them going forward. Sense the vitality in this movement.

Silently reflect on this mantra as you walk: *I am whole, I am complete, I am in flow.*

When you're done, take a few moments to reflect on your experience. What showed up for you as you walked? What was it like to be more consciously aware of the experience of walking?

As with any skill, learning to be an observer takes practice. The more you practice, the easier it will be to catch yourself when you get caught in autopilot, reacting to life rather than consciously choosing how you will respond.

Ride Out the Storm

When anxiety and fear show up, they can drain away your strongest resolve. It can seem nearly impossible to be inside your own skin and stay where you are. We naturally want to get away from discomfort. The urge to do something can be uncomfortably strong, having the energy and explosive force of an intense storm. This can leave you feeling out of control and frightened.

Still, most storms begin small, way out on the horizon. Some will move in and over you, unleash their energy for a bit. Eventually, they all move on. You can learn to ride out the stormy weather of your urges, to struggle and resist your WAFs by learning to ride along with the energy inside—the thunder of your impulses, the lightning of your fear, the relentless uncertainty of your anxiety, or the pounding wind and rain that drive your tendency to cut and run. You can practice just being with it, without letting it blow you away.

This next exercise will give you more practice getting in touch with this energy without automatically doing what it commands. You'll need about five minutes and a quiet place where you can listen to the audio at http://www.newharbinger.com/54476 and follow along.

EXERCISE: Riding the Storm Out

Get comfortable in your chair and allow your eyes to close gently... Take a few moments to notice the natural rhythm of your breath as you breathe in...and out.

As you settle, bring to mind a recent situation where you felt the strong urge to cut and run from your fear and anxiety. Take a few slow deep breaths and bring the situation alive in your mind as best you can... Where were you?... Who else was there?... What happened?... What did you experience then, and what are you experiencing again right now?

As you bring the situation to mind, you may notice the storm of anxiety or fear rolling in. You can hear the thunder, or even feel the rumble of physical sensations. Notice any stormy physical changes in your body, including pain, pressure, or any other scary sensation that is kicking up and blowing around. There may be lightning strikes of thoughts, perhaps about your sensations and feelings. What's your mind telling you about them?... About the situation?... About you?

Next, bring your attention to the physical experience of the urge to act. Notice the wild energy there, as the pounding rain tries to wash away your resolve and all that you care about... Is there pressure, tightness, or tension? If so, where is it located? Does it have a shape?... A color?

Now, choose to ride the storm out... Imagine opening up, arms wide open, and staying with the wild energy below the surface of your experience. If you can, go ahead and open your arms as wide as you know how. This time you're not doing what you've always done. Look deeply into your experience without trying to fix it, fight it, or suppress it, and without acting on it. Find the pain and hurt driving the storm to new heights... Gently look at it, breathe with it, and bring kindness to it...ride it and let it be. Notice how the storm is trying to throw you offtrack and push you to act in unhelpful ways... Just stay there, your arms still wide open, bringing kindness and curiosity to the energy and pain, as you would do for a dear friend or loved one who is in pain and needs your help.

See if you can notice as the storm front within you starts to move on. Notice as things begin to quiet down and become still. And, as you rest in that stillness, notice what is new or different for you... See if you can connect with having done something good for yourself...your life...even if you were scared, feeling the strong urge to run or lash out.

As this time for practice comes to an end, acknowledge and honor the step you took with this exercise and commit to practice riding out your difficult urges in the service of your life. When you hear the bell, bring yourself back to the present and slowly open your eyes. Take a moment to reflect on what you've experienced and learned.

After a week or two of practicing mind watching, mindful walking, and riding out difficult urges, you'll be ready to apply the practice of learning to observe your experience wherever you are in your daily life. So, look for ways to approach what you do in a more mindful way.

Anything that requires movement could be done mindfully. You could even practice being more mindful as you do household chores, like cooking, vacuuming, washing the dishes, cleaning, doing laundry, or running errands, or with hobbies you enjoy. In truth, anything you do, including simply sitting and doing nothing at all as you ride out a WAF storm, is an opportunity to practice being mindful and present just as you are.

The point here is to practice being mindful of the experience of movement with your thoughts, feelings, and sensations. In fact, you can put a note in your pocket or purse or set an alarm to beep every hour as a reminder to simply notice your experience just as it is.

LIFE-ENHANCEMENT EXERCISES

Many exercises covered so far aim to cut the fuel source feeding the destructive power of your anxieties and fears. These are skills that take practice. So, for this week, we invite you to do the following:

- Commit to making a centering exercise part of your daily routine.

- Practice noting when you get caught up in old anxiety myths.

- Notice when your mind tries to hook you, leading you to feed the anxiety wolf.

- Practice mind watching, mindful walking, and riding out the storm.

- Remember that your breath is always with you—come back to it.

- If you haven't been doing this already, slow the pace down and work with the workbook, so it will work for you!

THE TAKE-HOME MESSAGE

Recognizing how mind traps keep you stuck is an important skill. It's a critical step out of the struggle-and-avoidance trap. You can get something different out of your life if you're willing to learn to relate with your mind, body, and feelings in a different way. This is a choice only you can make. We hope that you make it now and act on that intention as you work with the material in this book.

Mind Traps Keep Me Stuck

Reflections:

- Anxiety myths are self-limiting and don't serve me on my healing journey.

- The mind traps that keep me stuck and feed my struggle with anxiety must be seen clearly and acknowledged.

- Learning to watch and observe my experience as I might a sunset is an important step out of the anxiety trap and into my life.

Inquiries:

- Am I willing to let go of any myths or unhelpful beliefs I have about anxiety and fear?

- Can I learn to watch my mind rather than be jerked around by it?

- Am I willing to stop feeding my fear and anxiety wolves?

- Am I willing to face what buying into my raucous and judgmental mind has cost me?

PART 2

Discovering What Matters and What Gets in Your Way

Your values create your internal compass that can navigate how you make decisions in your life.

—Roy T. Bennett

CHAPTER 4

Taking Control of Your Life

Life is a choice. Anxiety is not a choice. Either way you go, you will have problems and pain. So your choice here is not about whether or not to have anxiety. Your choice is whether or not to live a meaningful life.

—Steven C. Hayes

I t's hard to live a meaningful life when consumed with trying to control your anxiety. Every moment spent on this goal is a moment away from living your life in ways that are meaningful to you.

Take this moment to reflect on what truly matters to you. Are your choices aligned with your values and what makes life meaningful to you? Or are you driven by anxiety and the need for control?

Often, anxiety controls our lives when we prioritize avoidance over our values. It's time to change this pattern. Instead of feeding your anxiety, you will start feeding your heart's deepest longings and desires. This shift, along with applying mindful acceptance and compassion for your experiences, will prevent anxiety from taking over, and allow you to reclaim your power to choose a different direction.

In this chapter and the next, you'll discover, or perhaps rediscover, what's important to you. This is a moment to take stock. Look around the edges. Look for places where your mind may be feeding you the same old false hope. Perhaps in the back of your mind you're still holding on to the idea that you can make anxiety go away. If you find yourself still stuck in this waiting place, then reflect on the following questions before moving on:

1. Are my choices aligned with my values and what I deeply care about in life?

2. Am I engaging in activities that bring meaning and fulfillment to my life?

3. Or are my decisions motivated by the desire to avoid anxiety and maintain control?

Often people who struggle with anxiety answer no to the first and second question, and yes to the third. Translated, this means that anxiety is controlling your life, not you. This is what needs to change.

EXERCISE: Life Without Acting on WAFs

Consider how your life would change without constantly battling your worries, anxieties, and fears, or WAFs. Picture yourself engaging in activities that bring joy and fulfillment. Reflect on how your relationships might evolve in this scenario.

Go ahead, sit back, close your eyes, and take a moment or two to center yourself as you've done before. Take a moment to imagine your ideal life and note your thoughts below.

_____

_____

_____

Review your reflections and consider if they highlight important aspects of life that have been over-shadowed by your WAFs. We'd like you to reconnect with these aspects, because they represent your values. Let's have a closer look.

DEFINING YOUR VALUES

When we speak of values, we're not talking about your morals, beliefs, or philosophy—whether what you believe is right or wrong, just, or true. When we refer to your values, we mean two things. First, what matters most to you and only you! And second, what you do in your life to express what matters most. The second piece is critical because your values find expression in your actions.

So, you may believe that you should be a good parent, but without any actions, your belief is just that—a bunch of thoughts swirling around in your head. If you want to move that belief into values, then you'll need to look at your actions in your role as parent. You might even ask, *What do I do to express my value of being a good parent? What does that look like?* Likewise, if you believe in helping others, you need to act in helpful ways. If you don't live out your values, they're just empty beliefs. Beliefs or morality without action are dead ends.

So, to answer the question "What are my values?" you need to allow yourself time to think about areas of your life that are deeply important to you and what you want to be about as a person in those areas. These are the things that make your life worth living, that you cherish and nurture, and that you'd act to defend if necessary. By completing the exercises in this chapter and the next, you'll get a very clear sense of what *you* value.

Values Are Like a Beacon in the WAF Storm

Values are like a lighthouse, guiding you through life's storms and toward what truly matters. They empower you to navigate challenges and move forward, regardless of the circumstances. Without values, you'll end up like the person in the image below—stuck.

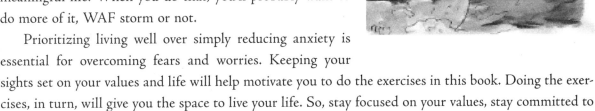

You know that your WAFs come and go just like the weather. Sometimes they're strong, sometimes weak, sometimes surprising, and at other times predictable. Other thoughts and feelings do this too. Unlike fleeting emotions, values remain constant, offering stability amidst change. By identifying and nurturing your values, you pave the way for a meaningful life. When you do that, you'll probably want to do more of it, WAF storm or not.

Prioritizing living well over simply reducing anxiety is essential for overcoming fears and worries. Keeping your sights set on your values and life will help motivate you to do the exercises in this book. Doing the exercises, in turn, will give you the space to live your life. So, stay focused on your values, stay committed to the process, and you'll find the freedom to live authentically.

We know that this isn't easy. We also know you can do it.

Live Your Values or Struggle with Anxiety

The choices we face boil down to living our values or living to avoid pain, difficulty, and the very real human potential for suffering. Knowing your values is crucial in making such decisions, especially when feeling anxious or worried.

Values are your benchmark for deciding which actions are useful and which are not. This is especially important when you feel anxious, worried, or panicky and wonder what to do. At those times, you know from experience that your mind will put you in overdrive, feeding you all kinds of "solutions" that haven't really worked. Even now, you may still feel the pull of your old history: *Listen to us… Give us one more go… Maybe it'll work this time.* In those moments, it's critical to focus on and listen to your values.

When WAFs grip you, ask, *Does this choice or action move me toward or away from my values?* Your answer will help you move forward instead of resorting to ineffective strategies. It's the intention behind your actions that matters. For example, someone may work long hours because it aligns with their values of purpose and contribution, while another may use work to escape from life's challenges. Values provide direction and help prioritize how you use your time and resources.

PROBLEMS FINDING VALUES

We've found that some people have problems identifying their values. At times, they also confuse values with goals or have a hard time separating values from feelings. If left unchecked, these and other concerns can keep you stuck. We'll briefly discuss some common issues in case they come up for you.

"I Don't Have Any!"

Sometimes we hear people say they don't have any values. When we ask more questions, they discover that they do have values but feel overwhelmed by WAF barriers.

Doug is one of many people who struggled with this problem. For much of his life, he suffered from obsessive-compulsive problems and excessive worrying. He told us, "I don't really care anymore about friends and intimate relationships. Every time I try to get close to people, I feel like they just push me away. I've gone out on some first dates in the past, but it never works out. None of my first dates turn into second dates or a long-term relationship. I think potential partners aren't into me because of my weird habits."

Despite his social struggles, Doug's pain hinted at underlying values. In fact, there'd be no reason for him to feel badly about missing social connection if he didn't care about his social life. Reframing the question from "Can I achieve this?" to "Do I care about this?" helped him identify his values. You can ask yourself this question too.

Doug was thinking about his values in terms of goals and social outcomes, like having a girlfriend. With some work, Doug acknowledged that he could not control having a girlfriend, because if he could, he would have one right away. He then began considering steps to support his social values, recognizing that deep connections take time to form and may not materialize right away.

Focusing on Future Outcomes

Doug fell into the trap of viewing values as a means to achieve future outcomes. *If I do this or that now, then I will get this or that in the future.*

Value-focused living is about embracing the journey, not fixating on results. Destinations are the steps you take along the way to creating a life. Like any journey, you can't predict the exact outcomes of your actions. Outcomes—good, bad, and sometimes ugly—will not be known until after you step. And even then, they need not diminish the value that guided you in taking the journey in the first place. The point of valuing is that you do what's most important to you in your life. And you do it in the here and now. You also do it because you care. It's not about outcomes.

Parenting exemplifies this uncertainty—parents strive for the best for their children without knowing the future. The same is true of other values. In the moment you don't know how things will turn out.

Still, it's so easy to get stuck setting goals to get the result you want. In a way we're always looking into the unknown future and miss the moment-to-moment process and sweetness of engaging our values right here, right now. If you choose values solely based on results and outcomes, you're living in the uncertain future. And you'll likely be disappointed if things don't work out as hoped.

This is why the essence of valuing lies in the present moment, focusing on what's important to you now, rather than banking on future outcomes.

Following Your Head Instead of Your Heart

When identifying values, it's not just about finding the right words—it's about connecting with your heart and soul. Values are not a heady, intellectual thing. They're about your gut, heart, soul, and spirit. So, when exploring your values and goals, listen to your heart rather than blindly following your mind.

Sometimes people express values and goals without genuine enthusiasm, merely because they feel they should. It's crucial to ask yourself, *Is this truly important to me, or am I doing it out of obligation?* Here, watch for words like "should," "must," "ought," and "have to" as signaling that your values may not be your own, in that they don't flow from your heart and deepest longings.

When faced with choices between comfort and what truly matters, anxiety and fear often push for comfort and relative safety. To break this cycle, you must desire something more deeply. As we move on, we'll help you clarify what that something is and how much you truly want it.

Choosing Values That Aren't Yours

Sometimes people don't freely choose values but choose ones that sound socially appropriate, make them look good, or meet others' expectations of them. Take the value of being considerate of others. Other people may expect that of you, but do you really care about it? Even if you do have roles and obligations, you can still connect with the values behind what you do and make it a choice instead of a should or a must.

So be sure that your values are *your* values, not values that society, friends, or family impose on you. Ask yourself, *Why am I doing this? Am I doing this because I care about it? Or am I doing it for someone else or to avoid someone else being hurt or disappointed by my choices?*

Remember, values are about discovering or rediscovering what's truly important in your own life—what *you* want your life to stand for, not what other people want from you or for you. If you turn your values over to someone else, you won't get to live your life.

Not Knowing If You're Heading the Right Way

Moving toward your important values can invigorate you, even if each step doesn't feel great. Sometimes you'll experience vitality as you take a step, but other times you won't. This is true for many worthwhile activities that require effort and perseverance.

Just think of something you care about in life and important things you've done in the service of that important value. You've probably had many "not feeling great at the time" steps along the way. Yet you have persisted because, when you look back at your steps against the backdrop of your values, you can say, "Yes, my actions are part of something bigger. They leave me feeling more satisfied and alive at the end of the day." When you can say that, you've found a value and a goal that really strikes a chord in you.

Consider the hard work you're doing to improve your life by reading this book—a value of health and wellness. While it may not always feel easy, each step aligns with your overarching values, leaving you feeling more satisfied and alive.

Goals can help propel you toward your values, but it's essential to assess each activity's vitality against your values. If a goal doesn't enhance your sense of vitality, reassess it and adjust course. Keeping your values in sight ensures you're moving in the right direction.

Is It a Goal or a Value?

Values are not the same as goals. Goals are specific tasks or achievements that can be completed and checked off a list, such as taking out the garbage or getting married. The same is true of goals like going on vacation, earning a degree, or mowing the lawn.

In contrast, values are a lifelong journey that guide you throughout your life and have no endpoint.

> *You cannot ever finish a value.*

For instance, getting married is a goal, but being a loving, devoted partner is a value that requires continuous effort and growth. Values like being a loving person or a good parent manifest in your day-to-day actions and are ongoing commitments.

When considering your values, you'll never be able to say "I finished that." Still, your goals move you forward along the journey and embody its purpose.

To uncover the values underlying your goals, ask yourself why the goal is important to you and where it fits into the bigger picture of your life. Answers to these questions will point toward your values. They'll also change the way you look at things. This perspective shift can transform seemingly mundane tasks, like taking out the garbage, into meaningful expressions of your values such as helping, caring for the environment, or being a supportive partner. It's no longer a stinky "have to do it" task. Taking out the garbage with an eye on your values changes the act of taking out the garbage. See if you notice that the next time you take out your trash.

Valuing How You Feel Rather Than What You Do

Many people assume that valuing depends on how they *feel* about an area in their lives. This is another trap. Here's why. You do lots of things in life despite what you're thinking or feeling at the time. Breathing is one of them. If you waited to feel good or happy before taking your next breath, you'd be in serious trouble. Many other actions are like this too.

You probably go to work regardless of whether you feel anxious, sad, tired, irritated, worried, or happy. Or you may visit your in-laws even if you don't care for them. Suppose you value social interactions and feel anxious about talking to a group of strangers. Not waiting to feel less anxious means that you can talk to them regardless of how you feel inside. Or if you're feeling panicky while attending a ball game with your kids, you can remain in the stadium even though you feel like heading for the closest exit.

Put simply, values depend on what you spend your time doing, not what you think and feel about what you're doing. This is why we emphasize that valuing is about behavior. You value with your hands, feet, and mouth (that is, by what you say). You do it despite how you *feel* about it. Many research studies have shown that if you focus on your actions, your feelings will eventually follow and take care of themselves.

Confusing Values with Emotional States and Traits

When people share what's important to them, they often mention desires like feeling better, more confident, and motivated. These seem like values, but they're actually emotional goals—different types of feelings and traits—disguised as values. Being calmer and happier are emotional outcomes too. You could even tick them off when they show up.

Emotional states or traits are outcomes that may or may not occur after aligning with your values. Remember, you can't control your thoughts, feelings, or how others respond to you in any reliable way. You can only control what you do.

Relying on emotions as the basis for action—doing things just to feel better—sets you up for disappointment. Chances are good that you'll *sometimes* feel better about yourself and generally more satisfied once you start moving in the direction of your values. But, no matter what you do, you won't always feel good, calm, confident, motivated, or accepted. Worse, if you wait to feel better before you take a step, you may be waiting a very long time.

Feelings are fickle. They come and go. That's why they cannot serve as a solid foundation for your actions. Instead, focus on actions that align with your values, which provide a stable foundation for meaningful choices.

YOU'RE AT A CROSSROAD

Right now, you're at a critical crossroad. You can either align your life with your deepest desires or continue struggling with WAFs. The choice is yours.

Let's explore how Maggie faced this decision.

■ *Maggie's Story*

Maggie came to us struggling with a major dilemma. Her daughter called to announce that she was pregnant and Maggie was going to be a grandmother. Maggie was thrilled. You could see the love on Maggie's face as she shared the news. She wanted to be there for her daughter during labor and delivery. She beamed when talking about holding her newborn grandchild for the first time. But then her tone shifted, and she became sullen.

Maggie shared that her daughter lives halfway around the world. In that moment it was like the wind had been knocked out of her sails. She acknowledged having the means to buy a plane ticket and followed with "But I'm terrified of flying." She hadn't flown in a plane in nearly thirty years. Just the thought of flying made her heart race and left her feeling queasy and nauseous. As much as she wanted to go and share the love and joy of her grandchild's birth, she didn't see any way to do that, because of her fear.

It was at this point that Maggie remembered the value question we talked about. And focusing on this question helped her resolve her dilemma. She knew that listening to her fear of flying was not what she wanted to be about. Instead, she connected with her values and the love for her daughter and the joy of holding her grandchild. And with that, she made a courageous choice.

She booked a roundtrip ticket and got on the plane with her fear. She said she imagined putting her fear in the plane seat next to her, and then shifted her focus to the joy of being with her daughter on this momentous occasion. Once back home, she relayed that her trip was fantastic. She also acknowledged that she felt quite anxious on and off during her flights. With a smirk, she added that she looked at her fear sitting next to her and reminded herself that she didn't want to let it control her anymore. In the end, Maggie didn't let her fear stop her from being the mother and grandmother that she wanted to be.

You're facing crucial choices like Maggie did. You could choose to live your life in alignment with your core values, anxious or not. A second choice is to say no to your life and retreat to relative comfort, safety, and avoidance.

You can think of these choices in this way. Imagine life as a walk down a long corridor with many doors. You have the power to choose which doors to open and enter. One door promises "no more anxiety," but there are countless others to explore in your life corridor—doors labeled "love," "fitness," "career satisfaction," "activism," and "inner peace." Which door will you choose? Reflect on past experiences. Did opening the no-more-anxiety door align with your values? Did this door let you move closer to your values or lead you further away from them? At this point in your life, you probably know the answer.

Now is the time to muster the courage to explore other doors in your life corridor. Think about your life. Besides the no-more-anxiety door, what other doors would you like to open? Maybe there's a door labeled "adventure" and another with a sign that says "creativity." There's a door to professional satisfaction and yet another is marked "growth and challenge." It's a long corridor with many, many doors.

LIFE-ENHANCEMENT EXERCISES

Incorporate these practices into your daily routine. Remember, acquiring new skills requires patience, so be kind to yourself:

- Maintain your practice of the Simple Centering exercise and any others you've found helpful.

- Take moments during the day to ask, *Is my current action aligned with what I value and moving me closer to my values, or is it a move away?*

- Reflect or journal about what living your values might look like.

THE TAKE-HOME MESSAGE

You can empower yourself by concentrating on what's within your control: your actions. Rather than struggling with WAFs, pinpoint what truly matters in your life and channel your efforts toward goals aligned with those priorities.

Your chosen values serve as a lighthouse, guiding you in reclaiming your life from anxiety's grip. They also help you stay focused on what matters amidst the clamor of WAFs. In those moments, pause, acknowledge your thoughts and emotions, and then heed the wisdom of your values. They will steer you toward actions that align with your dreams and aspirations.

Focusing on My Values

Reflections:

- My values illuminate my path, shaping my actions and defining my life for others to see.

Inquiries:

- Am I ready to let my values, not my WAFs, direct my actions?

- Will I prioritize living in alignment with my values above all else?

CHAPTER 5

What Matters to You?

We look for happiness in all the wrong places. Like a moth flying into the flame, we destroy ourselves in order to find temporary relief. Because we often find such relief, we continue to reinforce old patterns of suffering and strengthen dysfunctional patterns in the process.

—Pema Chödrön

What truly matters to you? This is a profound question we'll ask you to consider and reconsider throughout this book and for the rest of your life. It's a question that often goes unanswered until it's too late. We don't want to see that happen to you.

Here, we'll guide you through two powerful exercises: a funeral meditation (adapted from Hayes, Strosahl, and Wilson 2012) and writing your own epitaph. While they may seem daunting, these exercises offer invaluable insights into what you want your life to stand for. They also reveal what struggling with WAFs has cost you.

We all know that death is inevitable. Though we can't control when or how we'll die, we can control how we live from this day forward. We know from firsthand accounts that something profound happens when people have survived a near-death experience to live another day. Their lives change in dramatic ways.

Facing mortality prompts deep reflection and often leads to radical shifts in priorities. It inspires you to invest your time in what truly matters, leaving behind old habits and trivial pursuits. These activities are what you will be remembered for.

The following exercise will help you connect with this simple truth.

EXERCISE: Funeral Meditation

Go ahead and get comfortable. Imagine that you're observing your own funeral many years from now. Visualize yourself in an open casket. Smell the fresh flowers. Hear the soft music in the background. Look around the room. Who is there?

Perhaps you can see your loved ones, family, friends, relatives, coworkers, and people you've met at one time or another. Listen closely to the conversations and what they're saying about you. What's your partner saying...your kids...your best friend...your coworkers...your neighbor?

Listen carefully to each of them as they speak. Are they saying the words that, in your heart, you most want to hear about yourself? This would be how you want people to remember you. Your heart will let you know what you want and need to hear from them.

Now just pause for a moment and keep imagining this situation. Go ahead, sit back, and close your eyes. Stay with this image for a few minutes. Then come back to reading.

Remember the comments you heard as well as what you wanted to hear about your life. Take a moment and write down what you heard people say about you.

_____

_____

_____

Now write down what you wanted to hear about your life.

_____

_____

_____

Now reflect on what you heard during the meditation and what you have written down. Did people at the funeral always say what you wanted to hear? Their comments about you were based on what they've seen you doing up until now. Some of what you heard may have been disappointing. Perhaps one person said, "He was always so anxious and uptight... I wish he'd done more with his life" or "She had a tough life, never getting past her fears and worries."

The good news about this exercise is that your life isn't over. Your eulogies haven't been written. You still have time to do things to become the person you want to be. You can start living the way you want to be remembered.

This exercise was meant to increase your perspective on your life and your actions: you won't be able to see the costs of the anxiety struggle in your life unless you can see what you want to be about. Anxiety is costly precisely because it gets in the way of what you want to do. If this weren't so, you wouldn't be reading this book. You'd be just like the millions of other people who have their share of WAFs, along with other sources of hardship and pain, and yet march on doing what matters to them.

The next exercise may also seem strange and somewhat scary. If you stick with it and complete it, then you'll get in touch with what you want your life to stand for. So don't rush. Find a quiet place to reflect, openly and honestly, about what makes your life worthwhile. You may find it helpful to do this exercise in several sittings.

EXERCISE: **Your Anxiety-Management Epitaph**

Your task is to write your epitaph (the inscription on your gravestone) as it would be written if you were to die today. What would it say if it was focused entirely on what you've been doing to cope, deal with, control, or avoid anxiety, fear and panic, worry, painful memories, scary thoughts, and rituals? What have you become by living in the service of your WAFs?

Bring to mind all of your WAF coping-and-management strategies and how they've gotten in the way of what you want to do. Think of everything you say, think, or do to keep your WAFs at bay. Consider what you do before, during, or after your WAFs show up. List them all.

Here is what Jennifer, a woman with a twenty-year history of struggle with social anxiety and panic, wrote for her anxiety-management epitaph:

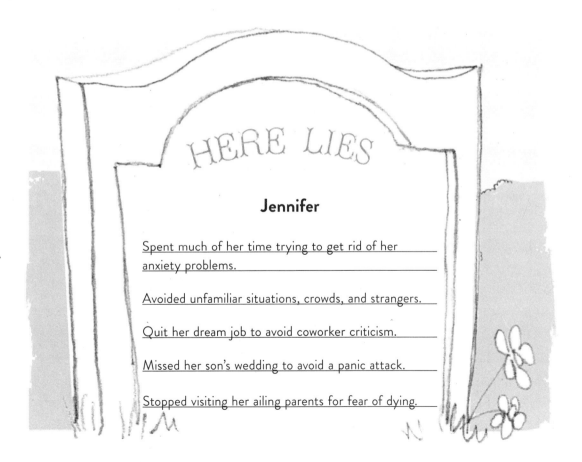

HERE LIES

Jennifer

Spent much of her time trying to get rid of her anxiety problems.

Avoided unfamiliar situations, crowds, and strangers.

Quit her dream job to avoid coworker criticism.

Missed her son's wedding to avoid a panic attack.

Stopped visiting her ailing parents for fear of dying.

Now, it's your turn. If you were to die today, what would your epitaph say about what you've been doing in your life to manage and appease anxiety and fear? Think about the costs and restrictions. What has happened to your life when you focus on not experiencing your WAFs? Write your own anxiety-management epitaph on the blank lines of the headstone above. Make it realistic. Start with writing your full name, and then use short phrases, as Jennifer did.

Next, you'll write a different epitaph, this time as you'd really like it to read, without the weight of anxiety and fear holding you down. This epitaph is about the things you truly wish to be known for.

EXERCISE: Your Valued-Life Epitaph

Imagine that you would choose to live your life guided by what your truly care about. In this version of your life, you still experience WAFs, but they're no longer a problem for you or a barrier to your life. Wouldn't that be something? What would you end up doing? What would you want to be about?

As you connect with this, imagine your epitaph. What inscription would you like to see on your headstone?

Think of a phrase or series of brief statements that would capture the essence of the life you want to lead. What is it you want to be remembered for? If you could somehow live your life without WAFs looming over your head, what would you be doing with your time and energy?

Give yourself a few moments to think about these important questions. If you find an answer—or more than one—write it down on the lines of the headstone. Add your name at the top. Think big. There are no limits to what you can be remembered for.

This isn't just a hypothetical exercise. What you'll be remembered for, what defines your life, is up to you. It depends on what you do now. It depends on the actions you take. This is how you determine the wording of your epitaph.

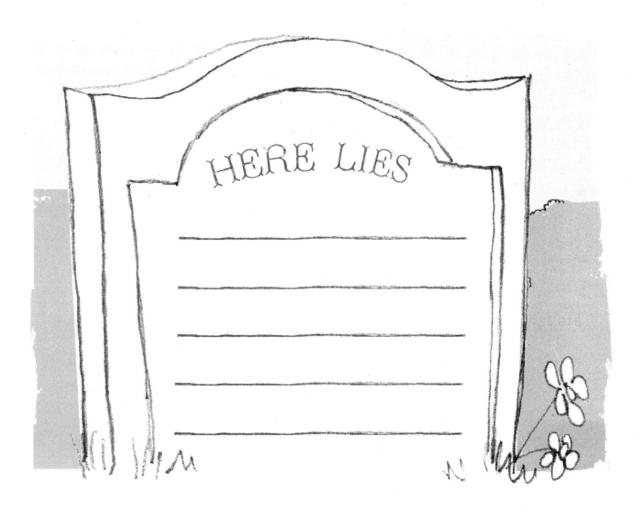

Of course, we can't promise that people will build a Lincoln-type memorial honoring you at the end of your life. Yet if you're persistent about moving in valued directions, chances are that people will write things on your tombstone other than "Here lies Tom: he finally got rid of his anxiety disorder" or "Here lies Mary: she spent most of her life struggling with panic." If these inscriptions don't excite you, you're in good company. We've done this exercise with many people, and no one has wanted to be remembered for their struggle with anxiety.

When you're finished, compare the two epitaphs you've written. You might find it helpful to print copies of both epitaphs, so you can compare them side by side and really look at them carefully. As you read each of them again, ask yourself the following questions:

- What epitaph do you want to be known for?

- Which epitaph leaves you feeling more alive, energized, and hopeful?

- What epitaph best fits your life now?

- Is your life about anxiety management or life management?

- Are your WAFs controlling you, and is this what you want to be about?

- What have you become in the service of your WAFs?

- Are you living better?

- Must you be free of WAFs to live the life you want?

We understand that getting a handle on anxiety is important to you. But why is it that people never mention WAFs in eulogies and on tombstones? Perhaps getting rid of your WAFs—a goal you've been working so hard to achieve—isn't going to matter much in the grand scheme of things. Think of it this way: every sixty seconds you spend trying to get a handle on your WAFs is a minute away from doing something that matters to you.

> *People will know you by what they see you do, not by what you think and feel about what you do.*

In short, the WAF struggle pulls you out of your life. If you're not doing things to be the type of person you want to be, *now* is the time to live the life you want and do the things that are most important to you. To start, you'll need to make a choice to do something radically different from what you've been doing up until now.

TAKE STOCK OF THE TIME YOU DO HAVE

Earlier, we asked you to envision your life as a book. Some chapters are written, reflecting your past experiences, while many pages remain blank, representing the future. Despite the uncertainty of when or how your story will end, it's easy to fall into the trap of assuming there will always be more time, another day. But betting on a tomorrow that may never come can lead to procrastination and missed opportunities. We don't want to see that happen to you.

Right now, you can estimate how much time you have left on this planet. Not long ago at a training retreat, both of us introduced this exercise and did it ourselves. It was a huge eye opener. The experience strengthened our resolve to make the most of the time that we do have.

Now, we invite you to do the same. The exercise is simple and requires a bit of math and a calculator. When you're done, you'll have an estimate of how many days you have left. With that knowledge, we encourage you to ask yourself, *How do I want to use the time I have?*

According to the Centers for Disease Control and Prevention, the average life expectancy is 76.4 years in the United States (Xu et al. 2022) and a bit higher in some other Western countries around the world, based on data from 2021. Though we know that women tend to have a longer life expectancy than men, to keep this exercise simple, we'll assume that we all have about seventy-seven years, or 28,105 days, to live our lives.

Now, go ahead and calculate how many days you've already lived by multiplying your current age in years by 365. Next, take that number and subtract it from 28,105. This new number is an estimate of the number of days you likely have left to live.

What number did you come up with? This number may be alarming to look at, but it's important that you keep it in mind. It reflects the time you may have to craft the story of your life from this point forward. So, again, how do you want to use the time that you have left? This is a choice you have control over, but whether you make this choice is really up to you.

This is a watershed moment. There's a lesson here that can change your life. Knowing in your mind and heart that everything you've done to get rid of anxiety hasn't worked is the first step on a new road. Embracing this truth paradoxically offers newfound hope—you're no longer bound by ineffective coping strategies—but what's next?

Start by trusting your lived experiences. Reflect on how your attempts to manage WAFs have led you to this point of feeling stuck. Accepting that traditional strategies have failed opens the door to new possibilities.

Look back at your responses to the earlier exercises and what you wrote about in your valued-life epitaph. Doing something radically new is hopeful because if you do that, you risk getting something new in your life. Everything you'll learn from here on out rests on this understanding.

All the old strategies for *managing* worry, anxiety, and fear lead to a dead end. They hurt you. This is why you need to stop them. If your mind protests against this suggestion, then look to your experience for guidance. It's time to let go of old, unworkable strategies. We know this is easier said than done, but don't worry, we'll cover in more detail how to do this as we move along.

To begin, you'll need to learn how to see your struggle with WAFS and its costs as they unfold, moment to moment, day in and day out, in real time. This is a skill that you can learn, and the LIFE Worksheet will help you do that.

EXERCISE: The LIFE Worksheet

The acronym LIFE stands for "living in full experience." It reflects our intention to frame this exercise in terms of what really counts: you living your life. A blank copy of the worksheet is at the end of this chapter and can also be downloaded at http://www.newharbinger.com/54476. Be sure to print enough copies of the worksheet for this week and carry them with you. You'll need them.

The LIFE Worksheet will help you get a better sense of where and when WAFs show up and, most importantly, what you do about them when they do appear. The LIFE Worksheet can be used to monitor and track WAF situations and triggers, related experiences you might have (thoughts, physical sensations, and behaviors), your willingness to have those experiences, and how your reactions get in the way of, or diminish, your capacity to engage in activities and experiences that you care about.

Fill out this worksheet shortly whenever unwanted WAFs show up during the course of the week. Don't put it off. If you delay, you'll end up with inaccurate information. Proceed as if your life depended on getting accurate information about your experience—and, in a sense, it really does here—which means doing the exercise as intended. Inaccurate information won't help you.

The LIFE Worksheet is short. Simply note the date and time of an unwelcome WAF episode, identify the sensations you encountered, pinpoint whether the dominant emotion was fear, anxiety, depression, or another feeling, and then rate the intensity of the WAF.

The next question asks you about your willingness to experience anxiety and fear without trying to avoid your experiences in any way. Willingness is a topic that we'll cover in detail soon, but for now, you can think of willingness as allowing your WAF thoughts and feelings to be just as they are rather than struggling against them.

The last section has fill-in questions about sensations and feelings and how you responded to them. Take your time here because your answers will give you a clearer sense of what you're sacrificing, each moment of every day, in the service of controlling your WAFs.

Make a commitment to fill out the LIFE Worksheets throughout this week. Don't do the worksheets because we said they're a good idea. Do them because you want a different outcome in your life. Make it a choice. Are you willing to do that?

If so, then start each day with the intention to complete the LIFE Worksheets, as necessary, throughout the day. When you do that, you'll be doing something new and different.

LIFE-ENHANCEMENT EXERCISES

At this point in the book, we hope you're gaining clarity about what truly matters to you in life. This week, we encourage you to:

- Make a daily centering exercise a priority.

- Review and refine your epitaphs.

- Take your time with this chapter, exploring the costs of anxiety management and control.

■ Using the LIFE Worksheet, identify how your battles with WAFs obstruct the life you aspire to live.

THE TAKE-HOME MESSAGE

Every strategy, every failed attempt, every plan or effort to control WAFs, has diverted you from what truly matters. You've been living your anxiety-management epitaph more than your valued-life epitaph. It's time for a change.

You can liberate yourself from the struggle. The answer lies in a place you've never looked before. It won't be easy or straightforward, but it's where real progress lies. It will also mean heading *toward* what you instinctively turn away from. You are capable of this transformation. The tools in this workbook will guide you, but you must be open to your thoughts and feelings without resisting them. This new path offers relief from struggle, losses, and failures. All you need to do now is to keep reading...*and* do the work.

What Matters Is Living a Full Life

Reflections:

• My actions shape my life, defining whether I live by my anxiety-management epitaph or my valued-life epitaph.

Inquiries:

• Is the toll of anxiety management too high for me and those around me?

• Do I desire a life beyond mere anxiety control?

• Am I ready to relinquish my role as anxiety manager and embrace a new direction?

THE LIFE WORKSHEET*

Date: _____ Time: _____ a.m./p.m.

Check off any sensations you experienced just now:

☐ Dizziness   ☐ Breathlessness   ☐ Fast heartbeat   ☐ Blurred vision

☐ Tingling/numbness   ☐ Unreality   ☐ Sweatiness   ☐ Hot/cold flashes

☐ Detached from self   ☐ Trembling/shaking   ☐ Feeling of choking   ☐ Nausea

☐ Chest tightness/ pain   ☐ Neck/muscle tension   ☐ Other: _____   ☐ Other: _____

Check what emotion best describes your experience of these sensations (pick one):

☐ Fear   ☐ Anxiety   ☐ Depression   ☐ Other: _____

Rate how strongly you felt this emotion/feeling (circle number):

0 ------ 1 ------ 2 ------ 3 ------ 4 ------ 5 ------ 6 ------ 7 ------ 8

Mild/Weak   Moderate   Extremely Intense

Rate how willing you were to have these sensations/feelings without acting on them (e.g., to manage them, get rid of them, suppress them, run from them). If willingness were put as a yes or no question, would you be 100 percent?

NO---YES

Completely Unwilling   Extremely Willing

(arms closed)   (arms wide open)

Describe where you were when these sensations occurred: _____

_____

Describe what you were doing when these sensations occurred: _____

_____

Describe what your mind was telling you about the sensations/feelings: _____

_____

Describe what you did (if anything) about the thoughts/sensations/feelings: _____

_____

If you did anything about the thoughts/sensations/feelings, did it get in the way of anything you really value or care about? If so, describe what that was here: _____

_____

* **L**iving **I**n **F**ull **E**xperience (à la FEEL wksht p. 222)

CHAPTER 6

Finding Your Values

Happiness is not something ready made. It comes from your actions.

—Dalai Lama

Many of us pursue happiness like a fleeting butterfly, yet it's not something to grasp but to cultivate. As the Dalai Lama teaches, happiness emerges from our actions, flowing like a river from knowing and living by our values.

To foster genuine happiness, identify what truly matters to you and find ways to integrate it into your daily life. Research shows that people who cultivate a sense of value-guided purpose live longer and have a happier life (Hill and Turiano 2014). So, by getting clear about your values, you may create the conditions for a more meaningful life and a longer and happier one too.

You've already embarked on this journey with your epitaphs. Now, let's dig deeper into your values. Identifying your own values is the crucial first step toward the life you aspire to lead. Don't be daunted—instead, ask yourself, *What is the essence of my life? What truly matters to me?*

It's okay if you're having a hard time coming up with clear answers. Below we'll walk you through some exercises to help you get greater clarity.

WHAT ARE YOUR IMPORTANT VALUES?

In this section, we're going to help you explore your values. First, you'll pinpoint areas of your life that hold significance for you—these are your life domains. These domains signify where you want to manifest your values. For instance, your career might be a focal point right now. If so, then we'll help you focus on your values related to the life domain of career. Be mindful that some life domains may not be important for you at the moment, and what matters to you may not conform to societal expectations, both of which are absolutely okay.

Once you've identified these key areas, you'll examine your values within each domain. Here, you'll uncover or reaffirm what truly resonates with you.

Yet, simply knowing your values isn't enough. You must also consider your valued intentions. Your valued intentions are personal expressions of your values in each life domain. They're about your actions—how you want to embody your values.

Take spirituality, for example. Two people may share this value but express it differently, such as through prayer or communing with nature. We also emphasize intentions because without a clear intention, you really won't know what to do. Intentions make your values concrete, personal, and actionable. This exercise requires time, but it's crucial. It's about making your values tangible and actionable in your life. We'll guide you through it, and you'll find it's time well invested. So let's get started.

EXERCISE: The Valued Directions Worksheet

Follow each step in sequence as you tackle the worksheet:

Step 1: Make Importance and Satisfaction Ratings

Begin by reflecting on your current life. Then assess the importance of each domain by circling either yes or no based on your personal sense of its significance to you. It doesn't matter how many areas you deem important. What counts is your genuine evaluation of what matters to you at this moment, knowing that priorities may evolve over time.

If an area is important, go ahead and rate your satisfaction with this domain on a scale of 0 to 3, as instructed in the worksheet. Trust your instincts here. A lack of satisfaction may signal underlying issues. It could be that something is hindering your ability to live by your values in these crucial areas. Recognizing these dissatisfaction points can be invaluable when addressing barriers in later steps.

If you consider an area unimportant, move forward to rate the next one. Proceed until you've evaluated the importance of all ten life domains. If you have not yet rated your satisfaction with any of the domains that are important to you, do so before moving on to the next step.

The following two steps pertain exclusively to life domains you've rated as important.

Step 2: Uncover Your Core Values

Now it's time to delve into your values for important life domains. In each domain, you have space to list up to three values that resonate deeply with you. This is your moment to pause and reflect. Dive into what truly matters to you and what you aspire to embody as a person. If you encounter any roadblocks, consult the Common Core Values Guide provided at the end of this worksheet. Then fill in the spaces with words that authentically represent your core values in each significant domain. Remember, values are not mere goals—they're guiding principles that shape your life.

You'll notice that we've limited you to three values for each domain. This constraint is meant to sharpen your focus on what truly resonates with you. You might list three values for each area, or perhaps just one or two. That's perfectly fine for now. Simply give it your best effort. Stick to a maximum of three different words that capture your core values for each significant area of your life.

Avoid choosing a value that mirrors the name of a life domain (for example, don't select "family" as a value under the domain "family of origin"). Rather, delve deeper into what aspect of family of origin holds significance for you. From there, you'll likely uncover other words that capture the essence of what matters to you (such as love, support, connection, or sharing). You might even find that "family" emerges as a value under work/career, as you consider how your job contributes to supporting your family.

You may also notice recurring words across different life domains. Pay attention to this. These common words serve as the golden threads weaving together the tapestry of your life. They encapsulate the true essence of what matters to you, regardless of context.

Step 3: Craft Your Valued Intentions

To finalize the worksheet, return to each important life domain you've identified and review the values you've listed. For each value, formulate a concise phrase or sentence that imbues your values with meaning, and write in the space provided. These are your valued intentions.

Your valued intentions should epitomize what you aspire to embody with each of your values within a specific life domain. They encapsulate your individuality and the essence of how you envision living your life.

Ensure that the phrases you devise authentically reflect your desires. They should illuminate what holds utmost importance to you for each value in each life domain. Here, listen to the whispers of your heart and the echoes of your deepest longings. If we could witness you living out your valued intentions, what actions would define your journey? Your responses encapsulate your valued intentions.

As you embark on this task, remember that your intentions should be within your realm of influence and control. For instance, expecting others to respect you is beyond your control, but cultivating self-respect is within your grasp. What does self-respect entail for you? Again, your answer forms a valued intention.

Last, steer clear of intentions containing words like "more" or "less," such as "I would like to do more..." While you can always adjust your actions, focus instead on how you wish to express your values. This empowers your values to guide your actions, especially when external influences threaten to divert you from your chosen path.

The Valued Directions Worksheet

1. Work/career

Is this life domain important in my life NOW (circle one):

YES = It's important to me   **NO** = It's not important to me

How satisfied are you with this life domain right NOW (circle one):

0 = Not at all satisfied   **1** = Moderately satisfied   **2** = Very satisfied

Reflect on your values and intentions

Consider the significance of work in your life, whether it involves a paid job, volunteer work, or homemaking. What does work mean to you, and what qualities do you seek from it? It may represent financial stability, independence, or recognition, or it may offer intellectual stimulation or the opportunity to connect with and assist others.

Have emotional or cognitive barriers hindered you from pursuing a valued career or volunteer position? Perhaps fear of failure or reluctance to leave behind comforts has held you back. Or maybe you perceive following your dream job as irresponsible.

Don't allow these barriers to thwart your exploration in this area. There are countless ways to infuse personal fulfillment into whatever you do. Keep this in mind as you envision your ideal job or how you wish to channel your energy, talents, and skills. What does that ideal scenario look like? If you had the freedom to pursue anything, what would it be?

Consider what you want your work or career to represent. What values do you wish to uphold through your professional endeavors—financial security, intellectual challenge, autonomy, recognition, or making a positive impact on others' lives?

My Core Values in This Domain	My Valued Intentions for Each Value
1. _____	1. _____
2. _____	2. _____
3. _____	3. _____

2. Intimate relationships (e.g., marriage, couples, partnership)

Is this life domain important in my life NOW (circle one):

YES = It's important to me   **NO** = It's not important to me

How satisfied are you with this life domain right NOW (circle one):

0 = Not at all satisfied   **1** = Moderately satisfied   **2** = Very satisfied

Reflect on your values and intentions

This section delves into intimate relationships, particularly with a partner or spouse. It's an opportunity to envision what you desire to contribute to such relationships. What kind of partner do you aspire to be within an intimate bond? What values do you wish to embody in this role—what do you aim to bring to the relationship, regardless of what you receive in return?

How do you plan to foster deeper intimacy with your partner? What sort of marital or couple dynamic are you striving for? How do you intend to treat your partner, or someone with whom you share a profound commitment and connection?

My Core Values in This Domain	My Valued Intentions for Each Value
1. _____	1. _____
2. _____	2. _____
3. _____	3. _____

3. Parenting

Is this life domain important in my life NOW (circle one):

YES = It's important to me   **NO** = It's not important to me

How satisfied are you with this life domain right NOW (circle one):

0 = Not at all satisfied   **1** = Moderately satisfied   **2** = Very satisfied

Reflect on your values and intentions

Whether you're already a parent, caregiver, or have aspirations for parenthood, this section invites you to explore your desires in this vital role. What kind of parent do you envision yourself to be? How do you plan to actively support and nurture your role as a parent?

How do you intend to engage with and relate to your children? Consider what actions your child would witness you taking to uphold your values and what others would observe. What aspects of parenthood hold significance for you, and what do you aim to impart to your children?

My Core Values in This Domain   My Valued Intentions for Each Value

1. _____   1. _____

2. _____   2. _____

3. _____   3. _____

4. Personal growth/education/learning

Is this life domain important in my life NOW (circle one):

YES = It's important to me   **NO** = It's not important to me

How satisfied are you with this life domain right NOW (circle one):

0 = Not at all satisfied   **1** = Moderately satisfied   **2** = Very satisfied

Reflect on your values and intentions

Nurturing your personal growth involves delving into yourself as an evolving multifaceted individual—emotionally, intellectually, physically, spiritually, and behaviorally. This journey often entails gaining a deeper understanding of your true essence, which aligns with the domains you've already explored.

Personal growth intertwines closely with learning. While formal education plays a part, growth and learning can manifest in various settings beyond the classroom. For instance, amateur athletes not only reap health and social benefits from their sport but also relish the challenge and joy of acquiring or refining skills.

Reflect on your own desires for personal growth and learning. Do you seek to enhance existing skills or to cultivate new ones? Are there realms of expertise you're eager to explore? Do you find fulfillment in acquiring knowledge and sharing it with others? Contemplate why learning holds significance for you and consider the skills, training, or areas of expertise you aspire to pursue. What would you really like to learn more about?

My Core Values in This Domain	My Valued Intentions for Each Value
1. _____	1. _____
2. _____	2. _____
3. _____	3. _____

5. Friends/social life

Is this life domain important in my life NOW (circle one):

YES = It's important to me   **NO** = It's not important to me

How satisfied are you with this life domain right NOW (circle one):

0 = Not at all satisfied   **1** = Moderately satisfied   **2** = Very satisfied

Reflect on your values and intentions

While human beings are inherently social, our preferences and priorities in social relationships vary greatly. Some people cherish a wide network of acquaintances, while others treasure a few deep friendships. Some seek a blend of profound and casual connections, while others find solace in solitude.

Depth in relationships encompasses intimacy on emotional, spiritual, or intellectual levels. Consider the significance and quality of your social interactions. Are social bonds essential to you? What kind of relationships do you envision? What personal attributes do you aspire to cultivate through your connections? Envision yourself as the "ideal you" in your friendships—how would you interact with your friends?

Reflect on your talents, passions, and any gaps you perceive in your social life. What sets you apart as an individual? What do you bring to any friendship? What qualities do you aim to embody as a friend? Consider what it means to be a good friend and examine how you behave toward your closest companions. Why do you value friendship? These reflections can illuminate your desires and aspirations in the realm of social relationships.

My Core Values in This Domain	My Valued Intentions for Each Value
1. _____	1. _____
2. _____	2. _____
3. _____	3. _____

6. Health/physical self-care

Is this life domain important in my life NOW (circle one):

YES = It's important to me   **NO** = It's not important to me

How satisfied are you with this life domain right NOW (circle one):

0 = Not at all satisfied   **1** = Moderately satisfied   **2** = Very satisfied

Reflect on your values and intentions

Why do you prioritize self-care? Why do you invest effort in maintaining your body's health through diet, exercise, and fitness? How pivotal is physical well-being to you, and how do exercise and nutrition factor into your life?

People pursue good health for various reasons. Some find joy in it, while others aim for success in physically demanding occupations. For many, adopting a healthy lifestyle is a form of self-preservation, ensuring they're around for loved ones in the long run.

Many of us carry scars from past hurts or trauma, causing us to retreat into darkness and self-blame. However, practicing kindness and self-care can be a powerful antidote. By extending compassion to ourselves, we can ease psychological pain and foster healing, even in the face of ongoing challenges.

How vital is it for you to cultivate self-compassion? How might your life change if you embraced acceptance and kindness toward your emotions and experiences? Do you actively seek opportunities to show yourself kindness, and if so, how? If not, how could you incorporate self-compassion into your routine, even if it feels daunting?

Consider what drives your pursuit of holistic health—both mental and physical. Each person's motivations are valid and diverse. What draws you to prioritize your well-being, and how committed are you to aligning your actions with this core value?

My Core Values in This Domain	My Valued Intentions for Each Value
1. _____	1. _____
2. _____	2. _____
3. _____	3. _____

7. Family of origin (parents/caretakers/siblings you grew up with)

Is this life domain important in my life NOW (circle one):

YES = It's important to me   **NO** = It's not important to me

How satisfied are you with this life domain right NOW (circle one):

0 = Not at all satisfied   **1** = Moderately satisfied   **2** = Very satisfied

Reflect on your values and intentions

Pause for a moment and consider your relationships within the family you were raised in, which may include stepfamily members. Are your family connections significant to you? Do they imbue your life with meaning and purpose? Consider the type of relationship you desire with your parents, caregivers, or siblings. Are these roles and connections essential to you, and if so, why?

Consider your unique talents and passions in this domain. What do you bring to these relationships, and what do you feel passionately about? Reflect on any gaps you perceive in this area of your life.

How do you envision interacting with your family members? If you have siblings or stepsiblings, what kind of sibling do you aspire to be? If at least one parent is alive, what type of adult child do you aim to be? Take this opportunity to delve into your aspirations and intentions regarding your familial bonds.

My Core Values in This Domain	My Valued Intentions for Each Value
1. _____	1. _____
2. _____	2. _____
3. _____	3. _____

8. Spirituality

Is this life domain important in my life NOW (circle one):

YES = It's important to me   **NO** = It's not important to me

How satisfied are you with this life domain right NOW (circle one):

0 = Not at all satisfied   **1** = Moderately satisfied   **2** = Very satisfied

Reflect on your values and intentions

We all possess a spiritual essence, whether we engage in religious practices, engage in prayer or meditation, contemplate life's mysteries, or seek to deepen our understanding of ourselves and our connections with others and the world around us. While organized religion is one path, spirituality often transcends the confines of religious institutions, places of worship, or belief systems.

Take a moment to contemplate your spirituality, unrestricted by cultural or societal norms. What resonates most deeply with you? Are there elements larger than yourself that ignite your sense of wonder? What mysteries of existence leave you in awe? Is there something, whether tangible or abstract, in which you place your faith? Envision the role you want spirituality to play in your life and how it would manifest. If fully embraced, what qualities would it bring to your existence? Delve into these questions to uncover your spiritual aspirations and intentions.

My Core Values in This Domain   My Valued Intentions for Each Value

1. _____   1. _____

2. _____   2. _____

3. _____   3. _____

9. Community life/environment/nature

Is this life domain important in my life NOW (circle one):

YES = It's important to me   **NO** = It's not important to me

How satisfied are you with this life domain right NOW (circle one):

0 = Not at all satisfied   **1** = Moderately satisfied   **2** = Very satisfied

Reflect on your values and intentions

We're all interconnected within various communities, such as our neighborhoods, social groups, workplaces, and different organizations. You may feel connected to multiple levels of community, including the importance of giving back through your time, talents, and resources.

Reflect on the significance of being part of a community larger than yourself. Do you feel a sense of duty or desire to make a difference in the lives of others within your community? Reflect on the type of person you aspire to be within these various levels of involvement. How do you envision sharing your talents and passions to enrich your community? What tugs at your heartstrings in this realm?

Caring for the environment is a pressing concern for many, extending beyond traditional conservation efforts to encompass the spaces where we live, work, and play. Reflect on your personal relationship with the environment and nature. Do you find fulfillment in caring for your surroundings, whether through landscaping, gardening, or simply maintaining your home or workspace? How do you enjoy connecting with the natural world, be it through outdoor activities or contemplative experiences?

Consider if sharing, helping, or reaching out aligns with your values, and if so, how you can express these wishes. Reflect on any perceived gaps in this aspect of your life and consider how you can contribute to making the world a better place. What drives your commitment to community engagement and environmental stewardship? What aspects of community and environmental consciousness resonate with you on a personal level?

My Core Values in This Domain	My Valued Intentions for Each Value
1. _____	1. _____
2. _____	2. _____
3. _____	3. _____

10. Recreation/leisure

Is this life domain important in my life NOW (circle one):

YES = It's important to me   **NO** = It's not important to me

How satisfied are you with this life domain right NOW (circle one):

0 = Not at all satisfied   **1** = Moderately satisfied   **2** = Very satisfied

Reflect on your values and intentions

The way you choose to spend your leisure time can significantly impact your overall well-being, which is why it's important to give it careful consideration. Leisure activities encompass a wide spectrum, both within and outside of work.

Play isn't just for children; adults too can benefit from engaging in activities that tap into their playful and creative sides. Consider the value you place on expressing your playful spirit. Do you relish opportunities to unwind, have fun, challenge yourself, or explore new interests or skills?

Imagine your leisure time exactly as you'd like it to be. What activities, interests, or hobbies would you love to cultivate and explore if given the chance? Reflect on how you nourish yourself through hobbies, sports, or play. What draws you to these pursuits, and why do you find enjoyment in them? Delve into these questions to uncover the essence of your leisure pursuits and their significance in your life.

My Core Values in This Domain	My Valued Intentions for Each Value
1. _____	1. _____
2. _____	2. _____
3. _____	3. _____

The Common Core Values Guide

Listed here are common values people find important to them. This list is by no means exhaustive, so feel free to add your own values. This list is a guide to help you identify and clarify what is truly important to you.

Empathy	Quiet	Kindness	Risk-Taking	Appreciation
Parenting	Admiration	Surrender	Action	Excellence
Inspiration	Beauty	Peace	Control	Challenge
Belief	Nurture	Hope	Gratitude	Self-Expression
Sacredness	Calm	Change	Learning	Accomplishment
Nature	Community	Fairness	Partnership	Faithfulness
Adventure	Contribution	Truth	Pleasure	Security
Service	Happiness	Power	Serenity	Enlightenment
Play	Relationship	Inner Strength	Invention	Encouragement
Fun	Equanimity	Reliability	Honor	Work
Order	Connection	Structure	Strength	Intellect
Spirituality	Passion	Self-Respect	Imagination	Planning
Humor	Patience	Friendship	Joy	Honesty
Wholeness	Thoughtfulness	Intuition	Rules	Dignity
Family	Love	Home	Leadership	Dependability
Consistency	Grace	Mastery	Laughter	Integrity
Support	Winning	Growth	Creativity	Loyalty
Health	Tradition	Compassion	Sexuality	Respect
Safety	Attention	Spontaneity	Courage	Understanding
Pride	Rituals	Wealth	Sensuality	Justice
Trust	Discovery	Vitality	Feelings	Self-Control
Freedom	Generosity	Independence	Openness	Curiosity

Use the spaces below to add your own words:

_____ _____ _____ _____ _____

_____ _____ _____ _____ _____

CREATING YOUR LIFE COMPASS

The worksheet you just completed is the foundation for creating a "life compass" (adapted from Dahl and Lundgren 2006). This compass gives your life direction—with it, you'll know where to go from here. The next exercise will help you create it.

EXERCISE: Building Your Life Compass

We've simplified this exercise into four manageable steps. Having your Valued Directions Worksheet handy will streamline the process of constructing your Life Compass below. You can also download a copy of the Life Compass at http://www.newharbinger.com/54476.

Step 1: Identify Key Life Domains

The Life Compass features ten boxes, each representing a life domain from the Valued Directions Worksheet. Additionally, you'll notice three smaller, blank boxes attached to each domain: one for importance (the "i" box), another for satisfaction (the "s" box), and a third box to rate your recent actions in living out your values (the "a" box).

Begin by revisiting your Valued Directions Worksheet and identify the life domains you marked as "important." Then, on the Life Compass, mark an X in the "i" boxes corresponding to these domains.

Next, transfer your satisfaction ratings from the Values Directions Worksheet to the corresponding "s" boxes on the Life Compass.

Step 2: Define Your Intentions

Craft a concise intention statement for each domain you've identified as important. You may need to condense the intention statements on your Valued Directions Worksheet into shorter phrases to fit within the boxes of the Life Compass.

Remember, intentions encapsulate your core values and should express how you aspire to live your life within each domain—what actions embody your values? Now, write your intentions in the designated boxes for each domain.

Step 3: Assess Your Actions

Once you've outlined your intentions, take a moment to reflect on your activities over the past two weeks. Were your actions aligned with the intentions you set? Rate the extent to which you've acted upon your values in each important life domain, using the following scale:

Y = Yes. Your actions consistently reflect your valued intentions in this domain.

S = Sometimes. While there are instances where you express your values, there are also times when obstacles or competing priorities interfere.

N = No. You're experiencing barriers preventing you from living out your values in this domain.

Write your ratings (Y, S, or N) in the "a" (actions) box connected to your valued intentions for each important life domain. Focus solely on your own perception of your actions over the past two weeks, disregarding ideals or external judgments.

Now, review your intentions and actions. Assess the alignment between your importance ratings (marked with an X in the "i" boxes) and your actions (rated as Y, S, or N in the "a" boxes). Identify any discrepancies where your "i box" is marked but actions are inconsistent (S or N). These mismatches indicate areas where you're not living in alignment with your desired values. Such inconsistencies are common among people facing challenges like anxiety or depression.

For example, if you value family (indicated by an X in the "i" box), but your action rating is low (S or N), it suggests a significant gap between your desired and actual life. Recognize these discrepancies as opportunities for growth and change, to realign with your values.

Step 4: Identify Your Barriers

Discrepancies between your valued intentions and actions often stem from internal barriers—anything that obstructs you from living according to your values. Use the signposts on the Life Compass to acknowledge these barriers. Revisit each important life domain and explore what stands in the way.

Break down the barriers into the following categories:

Thoughts and images—What recurring thoughts or images hinder you from living out your valued intentions?

Feelings—Which emotions impede your ability to take action aligned with your values?

Physical sensations—What uncomfortable physical sensations deter you from pursuing what matters to you?

Urges and impulses—What urges or impulses, such as avoidance, anger, compulsions, or substance use, obstruct your path?

For each life domain, jot down any barriers you've identified within the signpost boxes. This exercise will help you address the internal obstacles preventing you from living a values-guided life.

Your Life Compass

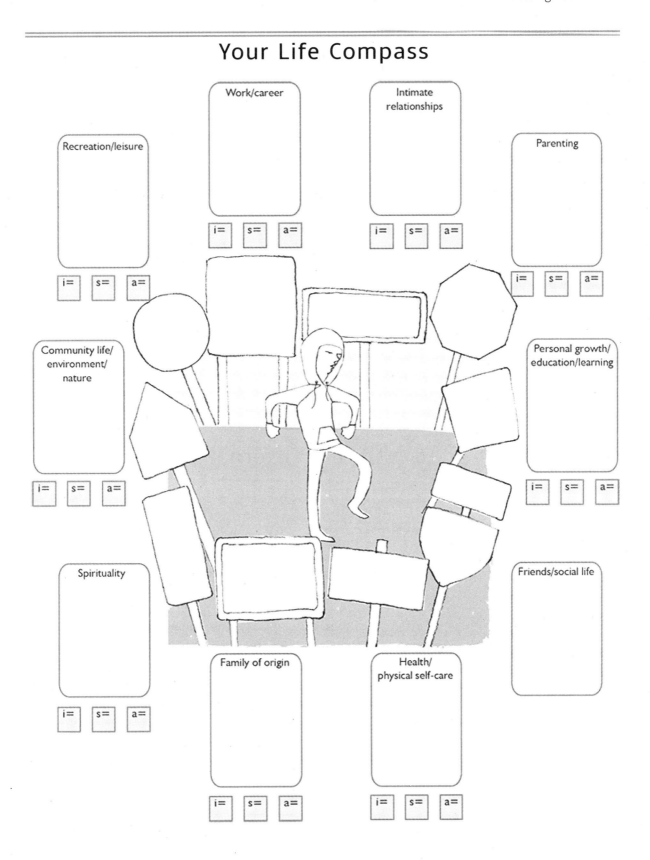

Work/career

i= s= a=

Intimate relationships

i= s= a=

Recreation/leisure

i= s= a=

Parenting

i= s= a=

Community life/ environment/ nature

i= s= a=

Personal growth/ education/learning

i= s= a=

Spirituality

i= s= a=

Family of origin

i= s= a=

Health/ physical self-care

i= s= a=

Friends/social life

Pause and Reflect on Your Life Compass

As you observe your Life Compass closely, you'll notice that many of your barriers are intertwined with your WAFs—those nagging thoughts, critical evaluations, judgments, unsettling feelings, and bodily sensations you'd rather avoid. These barriers originate from within you.

Anxiety about potential pitfalls and uncertainties can derail you from recognizing your valued intentions and taking decisive action. It's essential not to berate yourself for this. Many people grappling with anxiety encounter similar challenges and yet eventually discover new paths forward.

You also have the opportunity to leverage the insights gained from exploring your values. Let them serve as motivation to persist with this workbook, guiding you toward aligning your life with your fundamental values.

You might already have a clear understanding of your internal barriers, which is fantastic. However, if you're finding it challenging to identify them, the next exercise can offer clarity on the obstacles hindering you from living the life you aspire to lead. While you can read through the exercise, it might be more impactful to listen to the audio and follow along. You can download it at http://www.newharbinger.com/54476. This exercise typically takes about ten minutes and will provide you with a deeper insight into your barriers.

EXERCISE: Identifying Internal Barriers

Take a moment to close your eyes and center yourself in the present moment. Imagine you are sitting in front of a window, attempting to peer out into your life. However, you notice that the window is fogged up, obscuring your view. Despite knowing there's something precious beyond, it remains opaque and elusive.

Visualize each breath you take clearing the fog from the window, gradually revealing your valued intentions. Take it slowly, relishing the clarity emerging with each breath. Sink into this moment, embracing the vision of the life you aspire to lead. If it feels challenging, return to your breath, witnessing the fog dissipate as you gaze upon the person you aspire to be and the life you desire.

As you continue gazing outward, envision yourself living out your intentions. Focus on the initial steps you take as you decide to act on them. Notice your surroundings, your words, your actions, and the reactions of others involved. Take stock of your internal landscape. If the fog returns, simply breathe it away.

Observe your thoughts without judgment. Are there critical or discouraging thoughts? Notice any mental images or narratives that arise. Move on to your physical sensations—what are you feeling? If this is challenging, observe any sense of tension or withdrawal.

Identify any urges or impulses arising in your mind. Notice if there are commands to flee, react impulsively, or surrender. Acknowledge these without succumbing to them.

If anything remains unaddressed, observe it within your experience—whether it's thoughts, emotions, sensations, or urges. Refer back to the barriers you've identified to guide you.

Now, return to the present moment, sitting at the window of your life. Bring your awareness back to your surroundings and take a few deep breaths. Slowly open your eyes, with a clearer understanding of what truly matters to you and the obstacles standing in your path.

Using the insights gained from the imagery exercise, spend some time identifying and reflecting on your barriers. Recall past instances when you've attempted to align with your values, only to encounter obstacles.

These barriers could manifest as fear of experiencing a panic attack or other intense emotions; feelings of being overwhelmed, embarrassed, or vulnerable; intrusive and unwanted thoughts; distressing memories or images; worries about potential outcomes; concerns about failure or inadequacy; or other doubts and uncertainties.

Take your time with this step—it's crucial to gain clarity before proceeding. If you had trouble with step 4 in the previous exercise, you can return to the Life Compass and note your barriers succinctly, using just a word or two, in the signposts. Aim for specificity, as these are the hurdles standing between you and your values.

LIFE-ENHANCEMENT EXERCISES

Below are some activities that we believe will benefit you. Incorporate them into your daily routine and make a commitment to follow through as best as you can:

- Stick with any previous exercises that have proven helpful for you, and make a conscious effort to foster compassion and kindness within yourself.

- Dedicate time to deeply engage with your values and barriers. Use the Valued Directions Worksheet and Life Compass to guide you through this process.

- Begin each day by setting an intention to take action aligned with your most significant value(s). Be specific in your intentions, and remember that even small steps are meaningful. If committing to daily practice feels overwhelming, consider scaling back to every other day.

- When embarking on actions to support your core values, employ the skills you've been learning to stay present, gain perspective, and prioritize what truly matters.

It's important to acknowledge that these exercises may not always go smoothly, and any net positive changes may not be immediate or obvious. That's perfectly natural. Be patient and trust the process.

Consistent effort will yield meaningful results. Many people have experienced positive changes following this program, and you can too.

THE TAKE-HOME MESSAGE

Your chosen values are the compass guiding you through your life's journey, illuminating what truly matters. When worries, anxieties, and fears (WAFs) cloud your vision, pause and reconnect with your core values. A life well lived is not shaped by grand gestures but by the countless small actions aligned with your values. Your life story unfolds through the choices you make and the steps you take each day. Embrace the opportunities that arise daily to move toward your values, even in the face of anxiety. Let your values lead the way as you navigate life's twists and turns.

Identifying and Thinking About My Values

Reflections:

- Life's brevity underscores the importance of aligning actions with values, enriching my journey.

- A life consumed by anxiety's grip is not the narrative I seek; I yearn to embrace my life wholeheartedly.

Inquiries:

- What defines my purpose in this fleeting existence?

- Am I actively embodying my cherished values?

- Do I allow worries to obscure my path toward fulfillment?

- Will I prioritize living in alignment with my values?

- Am I prepared to pursue what matters, even amidst discomfort?

CHAPTER 7

Exploring the Costs

Pain in this life is not avoidable, but the pain we create avoiding pain is avoidable.

—R. D. Laing

L ife invites obstacles, problems, and pain. This universal truth touches every human being, often many times in a lifetime. Yet, in the face of adversity, the path forward beckons, demanding introspection and action. It's a moment to confront the toll of avoidance and inertia in the shadow of anxiety's grip.

As R. D. Laing teaches us, avoiding pain exacts a heavy toll, prompting the urgent need for healthier coping mechanisms. Your anxiety presents formidable barriers, yet alongside these barriers lies the vivid tapestry of the life you yearn to lead. It's time to face the costs of hesitation, evasion, and grappling with these hurdles. Now is the time for your life to unfurl its wings, unshackled at last.

This juncture is pivotal. With time ticking away relentlessly, many drift through existence on autopilot, neglecting to examine the essence of their pursuits, and pondering, *Is this truly my purpose, and is this what I want to be about?*

Here, we're inviting you to confront the consequences of your struggles with anxiety, acknowledging that it may be an arduous and difficult undertaking. Some of this may be painful for you to do, yet it's essential that you do it.

Roger von Oech, in his wonderful little book called *A Whack on the Side of the Head* (1998), likens personal growth to a sojourn through a junkyard, where relics of past desires and attachments lie discarded. This moment in your life is like that. It marks a departure from the realm of unhelpful coping mechanisms that you once thought were valuable.

As you begin working with this chapter, know that the choice to transcend your anxieties rests solely with you. We hope that when you reach the end of this chapter, you'll be willing to make that choice with unwavering resolve.

COSTS OF ANXIETY MANAGEMENT

Struggling with anxiety exacts a toll far beyond what meets the eye—draining your energy, stealing precious time, burdening you with regret that cuts to the core, squandering opportunities that could have been life-changing, robbing you of precious moments, imposing a heavy financial burden, constraining your freedom, fracturing relationships that could have flourished, and tarnishing the bonds closest to your heart.

Despite your earnest attempts to rein in anxiety, the bitter truth remains: your efforts have fallen short, leaving an indelible mark on you.

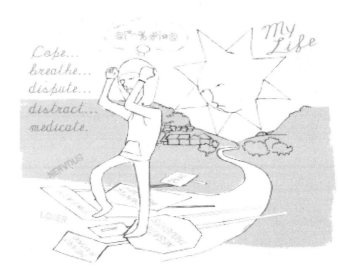

This is more than just a starting point; it's a critical juncture. It's about confronting head-on how anxiety has exacted its toll across every facet of your existence. Picture the sobering task of navigating through a cluttered junkyard, sorting through the wreckage.

Have you felt the fracture and strain in relationships, endured the onslaught of sickness and deteriorating health, battled relentless stress, faced setbacks in your academic or professional endeavors, struggled to maintain focus, or grappled with substance abuse as a coping mechanism?

Perhaps, in a broader sense, you've felt the suffocating grip of lost freedom, unable to pursue what truly matters to you because of formidable barriers imposed by anxiety. And there may be other costs lurking beneath the surface, ones you'd rather not confront.

The next exercise is designed to help you fully grasp the myriad costs of managing anxiety.

EXERCISE: **Costs of Anxiety Management**

1. Interpersonal costs

Consider the impact of grappling with your WAFs (worry, anxiety, and fear) on your relationships. Have your friendships shifted or, worse, faded away entirely? Do you find yourself distanced from family members, perhaps even driving them away unintentionally? Is there a palpable avoidance, whether it's from you or directed toward you? Has the weight of worry, anxiety, or fear led to the demise of a marriage or a romantic relationship, leaving you with heartache and regret? Or have you missed out on forging new connections, held back by the shackles of fear, dread, or an inability to trust stemming from past traumas? Are you finding it increasingly challenging to fulfill your roles as a spouse, partner, or parent, all because of those relentless WAFs? These are the poignant questions that underscore the toll anxiety can take on the fabric of our most cherished relationships.

2. Career costs

Explore how grappling with anxiety has derailed your professional trajectory. Have you ever found yourself compelled to resign or been dismissed from a job because you couldn't get a handle on your anxiety and apprehension? This encompasses instances of tardiness, decreased productivity, absenteeism, difficulty with travel, avoidance of tasks prone to triggering anxiety, abstaining from business and social engagements with peers and clients, or succumbing to procrastination. Have superiors or colleagues remarked on your diminished performance owing to your efforts to manage anxiety? Have these efforts blemished your academic journey, affecting relationships with educators and administrators? Have they ultimately led to joblessness or dependency on disability benefits or welfare?

3. Health costs

Uncover the toll on your well-being resulting from all the time and energy you put into dealing with your worries, anxieties, and fears. Do you frequently find yourself falling ill? Struggle to drift off and remain asleep? Experience moments where anxiety consumes you, leaving you feeling unwell or on edge? Are you hesitant to address your health needs due to your anxieties, such as avoiding medical appointments or necessary tests? Do you shun exercise for fear of exacerbating your anxieties? Have you found yourself making frequent visits to the doctor's office or emergency room due to your anxieties and fears? Explore the pervasive effects of managing your mental health on your physical well-being.

_____

_____

4. Energy costs

Explore the impact of managing your anxiety on your vitality. Do these efforts drain you at times? Have you invested significant time and energy into fruitless attempts at anxiety control? Are you frequently preoccupied with mental strategies to fend off or reduce your anxieties? Do you squander mental resources on worry, stress, and negative thoughts? Have you encountered challenges with memory or focus? Do you find yourself dwelling on past traumas or consumed by bleak thoughts about the future? Are you caught in a cycle of compulsive checking or rituals to ease discomfort or avert disaster? Have your efforts to manage anxiety left you feeling disheartened, fatigued, or depleted? Explore the draining effects of anxiety management on your energy levels.

_____

_____

5. Emotional costs

Examine the emotional toll of grappling with anxiety. Do you experience feelings of sadness or depression due to your worries, anxieties, and fears? Have you found yourself frequently on edge, occasionally erupting in anger during stressful moments? Do you harbor regrets and guilt stemming from actions or inactions influenced by your anxieties? How do these regrets impact your emotional well-being? Do you feel despondent or hopeless when your attempts to manage anxiety falter? Do you sense life slipping away while you struggle with anxiety? Delve into the emotional consequences of contending with anxiety.

_____

_____

6. Financial costs

Quantify the financial impact of addressing your anxiety-related challenges. Reflect on expenses incurred for psychotherapy sessions to address anxiety, depression, anger, or substance abuse. Calculate costs associated with medications, doctor's appointments, buying books about anxiety, audio or video resources, and seminars. Factor in expenses due to disability, lost wages, missed opportunities like cancelled concerts or travel, and absenteeism from work as a result of your WAFs. Aim to provide a comprehensive estimate of these monetary expenses.

_____

_____

7. Costs to freedom

Explore the constraints imposed by managing your WAFs on your ability to pursue activities you enjoy. Can you drive freely, whether short distances or long trips, alone or with others? Do your anxieties hinder routine tasks like shopping, taking public transport, or simply going for a walk? Are you prevented from trying new experiences, foods, or activities as a result of your anxieties? Does the specter of anxiety dictate how you structure your day, prioritizing avoidance of panic or fear? Reflect on how your efforts to manage anxiety limit your engagement in fulfilling pursuits.

_____

_____

Completing the Costs of Anxiety Management exercise is a critical first step in honestly facing how your WAFs have damaged your life and continue to do so. It's important to fully recognize the costs and actually feel their negative impact, despite your best efforts to change them. When you do that, you position yourself to do something differently.

WHAT HAVE YOU BEEN DOING ABOUT YOUR WAFS?

We've explored the costs tied to managing WAFs in your life. We've hinted at what makes them costly for you. But let's be clear: these costs have little to do with your WAFs themselves—they're linked to how you've chosen to handle them.

There's another option that involves a change in emphasis and a choice. Instead of struggling to control your WAFs to get your life back, you prioritize doing what matters most to you, even if it means facing occasional WAFs. Yes, it might be tough, but it's not just about enduring discomfort—it's about embracing fulfillment and living authentically. This is how you get your life back.

Right now, you don't need to fully grasp this concept. Your mind may resist, giving you reasons why this stuff doesn't apply to you. It may even tell you that we don't know what we're talking about. Don't argue with your mind, and instead consider two questions:

1. Have your WAF management strategies truly reduced anxiety and increased happiness?

2. Have they led your life in the directions you desire?

Most people answer these questions with a resounding no. They also know that the impulse to control anxiety and fear is hard to resist, even though it never works long-term. We don't want you to continue down the same path, especially when old strategies haven't yielded results. This is why it's so important for you to honestly assess your efforts to manage anxiety and how well they've worked for you. It's time to break free from ineffective patterns and pursue genuine transformation.

Successful anxiety transformation starts with facing each management attempt and assessing its impact. This isn't easy, which is why we've created an exercise to help you pinpoint what hasn't worked.

EXERCISE: What You Gave Up for Anxiety

This exercise aims to reveal the true cost of managing your anxiety, as you consider all the aspects of your life that matter to you, big and small.

Reflect on the past month and think about what you've sacrificed to cope with your anxieties. What have you missed out on or avoided in the name of managing your WAFs?

Write in the space provided under the two examples. In the first column, list the situations or events that triggered your anxiety. In the second column, describe your physical sensations, thoughts, and worries. In the third column, note the strategies you employed to manage your anxiety. In the fourth column, assess the impact of these efforts on your well-being. How did you feel afterward? In the final column, outline the consequences and costs of your anxiety management efforts. What did you give up or miss out on as a result?

Situation/ Event	Anxiety/ Concern	Anxiety Coping Behavior	Effect on You	Costs
Example 1: Was invited to go out with some friends	Fear of people judging me; was afraid of doing something stupid and embarrassing	Told my friend I was feeling sick; stayed at home and watched TV	Felt safer for a bit, but then lonely, sad, and angry with myself for being so weak	Lost out on good time with my friends; missed an opportunity to deepen friendships
Example 2: Was about to get on a plane with my wife and kids for a business meeting and short vacation	Was afraid of freaking out on the plane, having a panic attack, going crazy, being hauled off the plane in a stretcher, making a fool of myself	Got on the plane, but then my heart started pounding and I felt claustrophobic, so I got up and told the flight crew that we would be getting off the plane. We didn't take the trip.	Relief once I told the flight crew we were leaving, but then felt terrible and sad; felt disappointed in myself; embarrassed in front of my family	Missed an important business trip; missed what would have been a fun time with family; shame at hearing my four-year-old son say, "Daddy ruined our trip"—he really wanted to fly in a plane. Depression, loss of freedom.

Reflecting on Your Coping Strategies

Now that you've completed this exercise, let's assess what you've discovered. Have your attempts to manage your WAFs worked? Have they enhanced your vitality and ability to engage in life to the fullest? Or do your anxieties persist, hindering your progress and leaving you feeling trapped?

If you're like many people who struggle with anxiety, your efforts to control it always fall short. You may even find yourself regretting past actions, missing out on meaningful experiences, and sacrificing life's flexibility in pursuit of safety and comfort. As time ticks by, what does your intuition tell you about your history with anxiety? What lessons have you learned from your response to WAFs?

Anxiety and fear are powerful feelings that can overwhelm your strongest resolve. Despite your best intentions, you still bear the costs—struggling with self-doubt, avoiding triggering situations, and longing for change. You might believe that exerting more willpower is the answer, but consider your past experiences. Haven't you already traveled down that road, perhaps more than once? If so, then doubling down on effort alone isn't the solution.

EXERCISE: Are Your Coping Strategies Working?

Reflect on your coping strategies from the previous exercise. As you do, consider both obvious and subtle strategies like therapy, alcohol use, and self-help methods aimed at managing, reducing, or avoiding WAFs. Take your time with this assessment.

Be vigilant for strategies that offer short-term relief but hinder long-term progress toward what truly matters to you. Don't worry about strategies that genuinely contribute to lasting well-being and align with your values and life goals.

Distinguishing between effective and ineffective strategies can be tricky. Your mind may insist that a certain approach works and doesn't disrupt your life. However, consider this: What else would I be doing with my mental and physical energy if I wasn't using it to cope with WAFs? Answering this question honestly may reveal new, more fulfilling activities.

Here's how Alice, a twenty-four-year-old college student, conducted her cost-benefit analysis. Do your own assessment in the space provided underneath the examples.

WAF Coping Strategy	Costs		Benefits	
	Short-Term	Long-Term	Short-Term	Long-Term
Avoiding crowds	Can't go clothes shopping at the mall; feel bad about that	Keeps me out of many fun activities, like music, social events, movies; I feel like a loser	I feel less anxious.	Nothing comes to mind.
Distraction	Can't focus on much else; tend to miss important details	Becoming more forgetful; others describe me as distant, like I'm in another world	Keeps my mind off my anxiety; anxiety tends to go down, but not always	Nothing

After completing her evaluation, Alice realized that most of the benefits of her coping strategies were temporary and unrelated to her values and life priorities. They were all about getting some relief, even though it was always fleeting.

She also identified numerous costs associated with these anxiety management efforts. And she soon realized that none of her coping strategies offered any long-term benefits. Alice suggested that we consider eliminating the long-term benefits column because she didn't see value in it. But we've retained that column because we believe that you need to find out for yourself whether anxiety management and control offers you any lasting benefits. Take the opportunity to explore and find out for yourself.

PAUSING IN THE NOW

We know that working with the material in this chapter can feel heavy. Facing barriers and costs is challenging, but it's important to remember why we're guiding you through this process. It's not about making you feel bad; it's about identifying what works and shedding light on what doesn't serve you well. Without this clarity, you'll likely repeat past patterns.

Before wrapping up, we'd like to invite you to do another brief centering exercise. There's no right or wrong way to do it—simply follow along as best you can. This exercise is best done seated.

EXERCISE: Weakening the Power of Barriers

Go ahead and get in a comfortable position in your chair. Sit upright with your feet flat on the floor, your arms and legs uncrossed, and your hands resting in your lap. Allow your eyes to close gently. Take a couple of gentle breaths: in...and out...in...and out. Notice the sound and feel of your own breath as you breathe in...and out.

Now turn your attention to being just where you are. Just being. There's nothing to do but be in this moment, resting in an awareness of your breath as you breathe in...and out. Allow the sense of just being as you are to wash over you like a warm summer breeze.

When you're ready, expand your awareness just a bit and make contact with why you're here, working with this program. Notice the investment you're making in your life. Become aware that many other people, just like you, are also making similar investments in their own lives. Notice that you are not alone in this. What you're doing in this moment is an act of courage, integrity, and self-love. This courageous act of yours is united with many other people from all walks of life who are doing the same.

Notice any doubts, reservations, fears, and worries. You don't need to make them go away or work on them. With each breath, imagine that you are creating more and more space for them, more space for you to be you, right here where you are.

Now see if for just a moment you can be present with any anxiety barriers that come to mind. If your instinct is to struggle with them, just notice that, without getting tangled up in the struggle. See if you can allow those thoughts, and other aspects of your experience, to just be. Open your heart to them, and as much as you can, welcome them as part of your experience.

And as we get ready to close this centering exercise, gently ask yourself this: *Am I willing to learn how to change my relationship with my barriers and accept them as part of myself? And, are my life and my values important enough to me to be willing to do this now and perhaps again and again?*

Then, when you are ready, gradually widen your attention to take in the sounds around you and slowly open your eyes with the intention to bring this awareness of just being as you are to the present moment and the rest of the day.

LIFE-ENHANCEMENT EXERCISES

This week, we suggest the following:

- Make a centering exercise a part of your daily routine.

- Keep practicing exercises that resonate with you from earlier in the workbook.

- Take your time with this chapter—fully lay out the costs of managing your WAFs.

Embrace small changes, including the work you've done so far. They'll accumulate over time, leading you out of anxiety and back into your life.

THE TAKE-HOME MESSAGE

You likely opened this book hoping to find a way to manage your WAFs, so you can live the life you desire. It's natural to see your WAFs as the problem; many people do.

Our intention in this chapter was to help you connect with another possibility, even if it's challenging to grasp at this moment. That possibility is this: everything you've done about your WAFs has cost you more than the WAFs themselves. The struggle itself can be a trap, especially when you resist and avoid your own experience. We'll show you the way out.

Assessing the Costs of My WAF Struggles

Reflections:

- Life is a journey, not a destination.
- It's shaped by each small step I take.
- Spending time managing anxiety has come at a high cost and gets in the way of my life.

Inquiries:

- What have I sacrificed due to the time and energy spent managing my WAFs?
- Which has cost me more—the WAFs themselves or my efforts to control them?
- How have these efforts affected my life? What could I accomplish if I directed my time and energy elsewhere, away from managing anxiety and fear and toward my values?

CHAPTER 8

The Trouble with Avoidance

If you are facing a new challenge or being asked to do something that you have never done before, don't be afraid to step out. You have more capability than you think you do, but you will never see it unless you place a demand on yourself for more.

—Joyce Meyer

Thoughts and feelings of panic and anxiety are unpleasant, intense, overwhelming at times, and even terrifying. But as Joyce Meyer teaches us, it's avoidance that truly holds us back. It's the force keeping us from stepping out of our comfort zone, exploring our true selves, and embracing life to the fullest.

As we touched on earlier, research confirms that excessive avoidance is bad for you. Avoidance fuels worries, anxieties, and fears, and turns them into formidable life-shattering problems and possibly psychiatric disorders. Remember the image in chapter 1 of the person turning away from life and struggling with discomfort.

Toxic avoidance takes on many forms. Some people shun social interactions or avoid most situations where they may feel anxious or panicky. Others numb out with drugs and alcohol. We could go on and on, but here's the point.

A life of avoidance confines you, shaping your life around fear rather than fulfillment. It's a barrier that stands in the way of pursuing your passions, and it stifles personal growth. There's simply no way to approach your values while avoiding emotional and psychological pain.

EMBRACE YOUR BREATH INSTEAD OF RUNNING AWAY

Before moving on, we'd like to invite you to do another centering exercise to enhance the skills you've been practicing. This exercise focuses on returning to your breath, a constant presence that can anchor you during moments of anxiety or fear. This returning will help you when anxiety, fear, or any life circumstances threaten to take over and derail you.

Find a comfortable, quiet space where you won't be interrupted for five minutes. Access the audio file on the book's website or follow the script below. If you prefer, you can keep your eyes open, but fix your gaze on a spot on the floor in front of you to minimize distractions. We'll conclude the exercise with a gentle chime, signaling you to open your eyes and continue.

EXERCISE: Cultivating Presence with the Breath

Go ahead and get in a comfortable position in your chair. Sit upright with your feet flat on the floor. Place one hand on your chest, just above your rib cage. Then place your other hand on your belly, just over your belly button. Allow your eyes to close gently. Take a couple of gentle breaths: in...and out...in...and out. Notice the sound and feel of your own breath as you breathe in...and out.

Now turn your attention to the movement of your hands as you simply breathe in...and out...in...and out. Allow your breathing to be natural here, as you simply notice the movement of your hands as they rise and fall with each breath. There's nothing else to do, no state to be achieved. Simply notice and watch.

As you settle in, you may notice that your attention gets pulled elsewhere. Maybe you notice thoughts...thoughts about you...thoughts about this exercise. That's okay. When you notice your attention being pulled into your mind, simply acknowledge that, and then bring your awareness back to the movement of your hands as they rise and fall with each breath.

You may also notice that your attention is drawn to sounds around you, maybe sounds in the room or outside nearby. That's okay to notice too. Simply acknowledge those sounds, and then gently bring your attention back to your hands as they move with each breath in...and out...in...and out. Remind yourself too that your breath is always with you even if your attention goes someplace else.

There may be moments when your attention gets pulled into physical sensations in your body or even strong emotions. Dull ones are fine too. Maybe you're tired, or bored, or feel a grumbling in your stomach. The practice here is still the same. Gently acknowledge where your attention led you, and then kindly bring your awareness back to your hands and to the breath. Notice again that the breath is always with you.

As this time for practice comes to a close, let go of any thoughts and slowly widen your attention to take in the sounds around you. As you do, take two or three cleansing breaths in and out. With each cleansing breath, fill your lungs as much as you can with each inhale, pause for a moment, and then slowly exhale. Repeat one or two times, and then slowly open your eyes with the intention to practice bringing your attention back to your breath—your safe refuge.

AVOIDING ANXIOUS DISCOMFORT IS THE PROBLEM

Discomfort avoidance binds all anxiety problems together. While methods may differ by person and type of anxiety problem, avoidance remains a key coping mechanism and problem.

For example, those with panic disorder, specific phobias, and social anxiety steer clear of triggering situations—particularly situations where they've experienced intense anxiety in the past. PTSD sufferers avoid people and places that may remind them of past trauma, while those with OCD resort to compulsive rituals to alleviate anxiety brought on by intrusive thoughts and situations that might trigger them.

Likewise, you may avoid people or situations that provoke anxiety, avoiding activities like sex, exercise, certain movies, driving, unfamiliar or new activities, or certain foods. Coping mechanisms may help initially, but if they fail, you may withdraw or use various strategies to regain control—repeating positive affirmations to yourself, lying down, taking medications, sleeping, breathing, thinking pleasant thoughts, scrolling social media, playing video games, and on and on.

Let's take a closer look at how this unfolds for the people we talked about in chapter 2.

Panic Disorder

Jack's battle with panic disorder and agoraphobia gives us important insight into what people with panic disorder fear most. At the core, they're afraid of fear itself. For Jack, it wasn't cars or driving that frightened him most, but the looming threat of another panic attack and fear that he wouldn't be able to handle it. His need for safety measures, like restricting his driving radius and relying on his wife for support, eventually made him a prisoner within his own home. In essence, Jack's behaviors were about dodging panic attacks, minimizing their effects, or swiftly dispelling them. Likewise, his safety behaviors were driven by avoidance too.

Specific Phobias

As you saw, Avery's phobia of worms severely restricted her life and altered her behavior. Recall that she couldn't walk to work or be outside right after the spring thaw. She also worried about the impact of her phobia on her job and physical activity. While it may seem like her avoidance was solely to evade worm encounters, Avery understood that her true fear was about feeling sensations of panic, disgust, and nausea triggered by worms. Her avoidance stemmed from a deep-rooted dread of experiencing panic—an issue akin to those with panic disorder. Ultimately, by avoiding worms, Avery was trying to sidestep fear itself.

Social Anxiety Disorder

Carl's journey highlights that social anxiety extends far beyond specific social situations or public events. The core concern is fear of anxiety and discomfort in situations where others may judge him harshly. For Carl and those with social anxiety disorder, avoidance remains the primary issue. Carl's avoidance isn't solely about social situations, but rather he didn't want to feel fear and anxiety linked with the possibility of humiliation, vulnerability to scrutiny, or embarrassment.

Obsessive-Compulsive Disorder

Once again, the most troublesome aspects of OCD—the compulsions—are aimed at alleviating anxiety, tension, and discomfort associated with intrusive thoughts and images. These compulsions essentially amount to avoidance. Nathan's experience shows that compulsions consume time, energy, and resources, pulling you away from meaningful activities. In the absence of compulsions, Nathan would experience emotional discomfort and unwelcome thoughts, yet he would be free to explore and pursue other, more meaningful options.

Post-Traumatic Stress Disorder

The trauma may be in the past, but its lingering pain resurfaces at the most inconvenient moments. Within PTSD, much of the anguish stems from how people respond to traumatic memories, emotions, physical discomfort, and triggers. Sandra's experience underscores this truth. While memories and flashbacks are undoubtedly agonizing, they're not the core issue. Rather, the crux of the problem with PTSD lies in avoiding the emotional and psychological pain associated with reliving past traumas.

Generalized Anxiety Disorder

Samuel's life revolved around constant worry about work and many other things too. Despite his efforts to control it, nothing seemed to help. This ongoing battle left him drained and constantly on edge. What was hardest for Samuel to face was the reality that his worry was, in fact, his mind's clever way of keeping him from experiencing fear and uncertainty in life. Things do sometimes go terribly, horribly wrong, and no amount of worrying will change that. Avoiding this truth by worrying needlessly cost Samuel dearly.

YOU CAN RUN, BUT YOU CAN'T HIDE FROM YOURSELF

You can't avoid or get away from feelings of anxiety and fear, because the source of emotional pain is within you. It's not like you can get to safety by running away.

If a vicious dog were coming toward you, you could take quick and decisive action by literally running for your life. But unlike a vicious dog or any other external danger, internal struggles persist regardless of location. Traumatic memories and panic attacks can show up anywhere, anytime. You carry your thoughts and feelings wherever you go—they're inseparable parts of your history as a human being. If you're prone to having intrusive obsessional thoughts such as *I could have contaminated myself*, you know from experience that these thoughts can show up anywhere.

The bottom line is that your thoughts and feelings—the good, the bad, and the ugly—always go with you wherever you go. You can't escape or avoid your feelings of anxiety, apprehension, and insecurity by going somewhere else. You take them with you everywhere, along with everything else going on inside your mind and body.

Trying to run and hide from your WAFs is akin to trying to run and hide from yourself. There's really no way to do it so long as you're alive. To act against what you think and feel is to act against your very being. Resisting WAFs only leads to stagnation or exacerbates the situation. Acceptance, not avoidance, is key to moving forward.

You Can't Argue Away Your WAFs

Many people try to get a handle on their anxious thoughts and feelings by changing what they think, or by reassuring themselves, or by arguing with themselves. You probably know that this doesn't work well. You're right. So why can't you just talk your emotions away? The answer lies in evolution.

The oldest part of the brain, responsible for primal emotions like fear and panic, doesn't respond to words and reasoning such as "Don't be scared" or "Calm down." It's akin to dealing with primitive creatures like snakes or crocodiles—attempting to reason with them would be useless, even dangerous.

Similarly, trying to argue away unpleasant emotions is ineffective. Just as you wouldn't reason with a crocodile, you can't change deep-seated emotions with words.

You can't think your way out of feeling anxious or afraid, because of how the mind works. Each thought is interconnected, part of a vast network of connections. When you try to think yourself out of a thought, a memory, or a feeling, you must contact the very thought or feeling you'd rather not have. Doing so leaves you preoccupied with the unwanted thought and feeling and activates other thoughts and feelings connected with the ones you don't want to have. That's how the mind works. There's just no way to think yourself out of anxious thoughts or feelings without getting the very thing you don't want, while activating other unpleasant connections too.

EXERCISE: The Control and Avoidance Detour

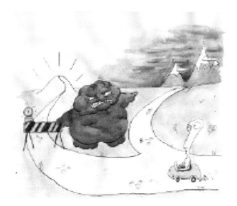

Picture yourself on a journey toward your Values Mountain, representing everything you cherish and aspire to be. It stands for everything you care about in life. You'll see it in the distance in the illustration on the left.

As you're happily driving along this road, anxiety unexpectedly appears, blocking your path. You slow down to avoid colliding with this obstacle, veering off onto the "emotional avoidance" detour as illustrated below.

On this detour, you find yourself going in circles, unable to move forward because the WAFs are still blocking the road. So, you go round and round, waiting, hoping, but going nowhere. It's frustrating. You feel like time is slipping away. This struggle with your thoughts and feelings keeps you trapped in a cycle of struggle and avoidance, preventing you from progressing toward your goals.

This is what happens when you struggle with your unpleasant thoughts and feelings. You feel stuck, going nowhere. You don't want your life to be about driving on the control-and-avoidance detour. And yet it's so easy to get stuck there when WAFs show up. In fact, many people get stuck there at times and for various reasons.

But there's another option. You can choose to take your unpleasant thoughts and feelings along for the ride. Instead of getting stuck trying to get rid of them, you can decide to move forward with them. This requires making a conscious choice to do things differently when faced with obstacles and being willing to accept and take your thoughts and feelings with you as you move forward. Otherwise, you'll remain stuck in the same cycle of avoidance.

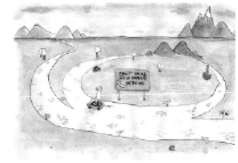

Even an impulse to act is a feeling. But the action isn't inevitable. There's a split second between every impulse and every action. In this gap, you can intervene to determine what you're going to do and how you're going to respond. The next exercise helps you get a better sense of this.

EXERCISE: Finding Fresh Options to Old WAF Impulses

Review some of your completed LIFE Worksheets. Choose one episode where the impulse to act on your WAFs was strong and where your choices and actions got in the way of something important to you.

Below, list the WAF feeling, what you did in response to it, and the costs of your actions.

WAF feelings (your thoughts, emotions, sensations):

_____

WAF impulse (your WAF coping actions):

_____

Consequences of your WAF response (what you lost or missed out on):

_____

How would you describe how you treated your WAF feeling and impulse (e.g., as an enemy, stranger, unwelcome guest)?

_____

Last, how would you describe the tone of your relationship with your WAFs (e.g., uncaring, unloving, unkind, loving, friendly, caring, supportive, kind, compassionate)?

_____

Step back and ask yourself, *Is it really necessary to act on these feelings (or this thought)?* What else might you have done instead? Instead of more avoidance, brainstorm some new and different life-affirming alternative actions. Write them down below.

Other life-affirming WAF responses:

_____

_____

Potential consequences of these new responses (what you would have gained in your life):

_____

The purpose of this brief exercise is to demonstrate that you have control and choices in this moment, regardless of how powerful the anxiety feelings and impulses to act may seem.

THERE IS HOPE—YOUR LIFE CAN BE DIFFERENT!

An extensive body of research confirms that avoidance is ineffective, costly, and can even make things worse (Akbari et al. 2022; Hayes et al. 1996). This conclusion covers a broad swath of strategies where the aim is to reduce, control, or somehow manage anxiety and fear. It doesn't matter how creative or sophisticated your avoidance efforts are. This isn't about effort or willpower. The hard truth is that avoidance doesn't work.

While this might be disheartening, there's a silver lining. Armed with this understanding, you can choose to do something other than avoidance. Embracing this shift will empower you to reclaim control over your life. The brief suggestions below will help you do just that.

How Do You Scratch Your Anxiety Itch?

You're not to blame for your anxiety troubles. It's not about trying harder; you've done what you thought was best. Now, it's time to stop scratching your anxiety itch.

How do you typically respond when anxiety and fear show up? How do you scratch that itch? Write down your thoughts in the space below.

_____

_____

Before moving on, reflect on how scratching your anxiety itch works for you. Short term, you probably feel better—it feels good to scratch a mosquito bite too. But if you keep at it, and maybe intensely, you may end up with a festering wound that becomes a much bigger problem.

What you need to do is learn to take care of your anxiety itch without scratching all the time, or getting bogged down in avoidance techniques. One way to do that is to do something else.

Become Mindful When Your Mind Beats You Up

People struggling with anxiety are remarkably resilient individuals. They're survivors. But they can also be very hard on themselves. They may feel inadequate, weak, or unworthy of a fulfilling life. They may think they're not trying hard enough or that they're somehow broken. This self-loathing, though not often discussed, is a prevalent feature of anxiety problems.

The judgmental nature of the mind can poison various aspects of life if left unchecked. However, there's an antidote—an escape from this toxic mindset. It begins with recognizing and intercepting self-loathing before it takes hold.

Take a moment to reflect:

What does your mind tell you about yourself and your anxiety? How does it beat you up? Jot down your thoughts in the space below.

_____

_____

Right now, you can start disrupting your unhelpful and highly critical mind by simply acknowledging the inner dialogue when it arises. Say to yourself, *There's the old inner critic again.* Later, we'll incorporate exercises and skills to foster self-kindness and compassion—an effective countermeasure to halt the negative cycle your mind creates.

Through these practices, you'll realize that your life isn't solely defined by anxiety. You don't have to persist on the ineffective path of managing and controlling anxiety or resorting to avoidance. Instead, you can learn to approach your anxiety differently. This is the hope and liberation we're after in this book.

Don't Believe Us or Your Mind—Trust Your Experience

You don't have to believe or understand everything immediately. Your mind may resist, labeling this book as too simplistic. But remember, your mind is not always your best friend—particularly when it tells you that you can't change and that you're really wasting your time. When these thoughts arise, don't get stuck arguing with your mind or trying to convince yourself of anything. Instead, acknowledge the inner critic, and see if its advice is helpful in terms of getting your life back. After that, move on.

Stay open to learning new ways of relating to your WAFs, engage in the exercises we've suggested, and observe their impact over time. Trust the process. Let your lived experiences guide you.

LIFE-ENHANCEMENT EXERCISES

For this week, we once again invite you to work with the material in this workbook by spending time with the following:

- Do one of the centering exercises daily or as often as you can.

- Track your anxiety and fear with the LIFE Worksheet (see chapter 5) and review with an eye on your avoidance moves, their costs, and experiences where you did not avoid but instead did something you care about with any WAF discomfort.

- Take stock of how avoidance plays out in your life.

- Decide to commit to doing something to support your values each day.

- When you're feeling unmotivated, revisit the costs of struggle and avoidance and then bring your awareness to your values.

- Continue reading and working with this workbook, but don't rush it!

THE TAKE-HOME MESSAGE

Avoidance is the common tie that binds all anxiety disorders together. Avoidance of fear and anxiety feeds fear and anxiety, and it shrinks lives. It's toxic for this reason. But we'll help you break free with compassionate actions and a newfound skill set that will uproot avoidance, allowing your life to flourish.

Discovering the Toxic Root of "Problematic" Anxiety

Reflections:

- Avoidance can turn normal anxiety and fear into a life-shattering problem.

- Perhaps the real challenge lies in confronting and addressing my tendency to avoid anxious discomfort, including trying to control it or make it go away.

Inquiries:

- What are some of the subtle and more obvious ways I avoid my emotional and psychological pain?

- Am I willing to meet my anxious discomfort with actions that are kinder, gentler, and more compassionate so I can lead a better life?

- Am I willing to say no to avoidance in all its forms?

CHAPTER 9

Ending Your Struggle with Anxiety

Experience has shown that, ironically, it is often our very attempts to solve the problem that, in fact, maintain it. The attempted solutions become the true problem.

—Giorgio Nardone and Paul Watzlawick

When you look at anxiety as a problem, it will naturally require a solution. Yet it's our well-intentioned solutions that are the real problem. Let that possibility sink in for a moment.

You've looked at how avoidance doesn't work and is bad for you. Unlike other areas of life over which you can exert some control, you cannot control anxiety. In this chapter you'll learn why. You'll also discover when and where control is effective, and how to shift away from managing anxiety toward managing your life.

ENDING THE TUG-OF-WAR WITH ANXIETY

Trying to control anxiety is about struggle. Letting go of the struggle means accepting anxiety as it is, without trying to avoid or control it. This is different from trying not to feel anxiety. You can learn to have unpleasant thoughts and feelings *and* distance yourself from them just enough to be able to engage in meaningful activities—whether it's socializing, driving, air travel, or enjoying entertainment.

When you let go of fighting against anxiety, you're not admitting defeat. You haven't lost anything either. Instead, you regain your freedom. You're deciding, perhaps for the first time, to surrender and to stop resisting your anxious thoughts and feelings. This is a smart move on your part, because defeating anxiety is unnecessary to have the life you want.

Surrendering involves four key steps:

1. Acknowledging the struggle

2. Allowing yourself to recognize the futility and exhaustion of the struggle

3. Facing the consequences of being stuck and limited by the struggle

4. Letting go to regain your freedom

Let's have a closer look at this process.

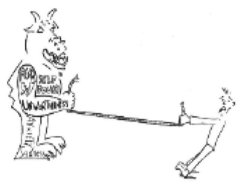

It might feel like you're in a relentless tug-of-war with anxiety monsters. No matter how hard you pull, they always return stronger. You've never managed to defeat them for good.

When you're locked in this battle, your options seem limited. You've got both hands firmly clenching the rope, and your feet are dug in, stuck in the same position. Back and forth it goes.

As the struggle intensifies, you feel increasingly overwhelmed—your chest tightens, your breathing becomes shallow, your teeth are clenched, your face is red with pearls of sweat welling up on your brow and forehead, and you can see the whites of your knuckles. You're stuck in an exhausting fight for your life, or so it seems.

Your options may appear limited. Yet you do have other options. What else could you do in this situation? Take a moment to jot down what you came up with.

_____

_____

You may have only thought of a few options, which is fine. Your mind might have suggested trying harder or seeking a new coping strategy or medication, but isn't that just the same old approach in a different guise? Old wine, new label?

How about this. What if you don't need to win this fight? Think about it. What if you simply dropped the rope? As you connect with this possibility, notice what happens to your hands and feet. They're free, right? You can now do something other than fighting.

To help you see how this might play out in your life, imagine someone or something you care about waiting on the sidelines—a loved one, a project, a vacation. They're watching and waiting for you to finish the fight. Would you continue the battle, or would you drop the rope and prioritize the person or situation that's been waiting for you?

Dropping the rope and ending the struggle creates space for something new in your life. Without being consumed by anxiety management, you open the door to pursuing the life you've set aside each time you've picked up the rope and engaged in the battle. As one of our anxious clients aptly put it, "When I drop the rope, I'm free."

WHERE ARE YOU IN CONTROL?

So why are so many people reluctant to drop the rope? Why do we cling to struggle despite its costs? The answer has to do with our beliefs about control.

As someone who struggles with anxiety, you're familiar with mantras like "Pull yourself together," "Think positive thoughts," or "Where there's a will, there's a way." But previous exercises and your own lived experience have shown that these strategies don't work with anxiety, fear, worry, and other forms of emotional and psychological pain.

Go back to the costs of anxiety management in chapter 7. Reflect on your efforts to manage anxiety. Have they made you feel safer or brought you closer to your desired life? Your experience likely screams "No!"

As strange as it may seem, it's possible to coexist with anxiety without letting it overpower you. How? By choosing to be willing to embrace anxiety just as it is.

You might wonder why control seems to succeed in many aspects of life but fails with anxiety and emotional pain. The answer is that anxiety differs in important ways from other problems in life that can be controlled quite effectively. Understanding this distinction is crucial, and we'll guide you through some exercises to recognize when control is effective and when it isn't.

You Control Your Actions

Action—or what you do with your mouth, hands, and feet—is a clear indicator of when control may be effective. Simply ask yourself if your actions and their outcomes are observable by you or others. Consider these examples:

- Want to tidy up your yard? Grab a rake and get started.

- Looking to change your room's wall color? Purchase paint and repaint the walls.

- Dislike some of your clothes? Donate or discard them.

- Unhappy with your job? Quit and find a new one.

- Miss an old friend? Reach out to them via call or text.

- Aim to spread kindness? Offer a gift, compliment, or hug.

- Prioritize your health? Exercise regularly and maintain a balanced diet.

> *I can control what I do with my mouth, hands, and feet.*

In each example, your actions directly impact the world outside your body. Controlling your behavior is effective in so many life areas, it only makes sense to apply control to manage emotional and physical pain happening *inside* you. Admittedly, at times, this works. For instance, you may take an aspirin for a headache, see a doctor for an illness, take time to relax, or exercise regularly to maintain emotional balance.

As we mentioned earlier, control in response to extreme traumatic situations—such as fighting, fleeing, or freezing—can be adaptive and necessary for survival. Imagine you're faced with a sudden threat like a speeding car while crossing the road. Here, the instinct to run or jump out of the way helps you avoid severe injury or death. This fear-driven response is a form of control that serves a valuable purpose.

Control can often become problematic, however, when we apply external methods to internal struggles. You may attempt to handle your thoughts and feelings as you would discard unwanted clothes. But can you simply dispose of your unpleasant thoughts and feelings like a pair of jeans you no longer like? Has that approach ever worked for you? Can you replace an old painful memory with a new one? Have you ever been able to do that?

Reflecting on your experiences ought to show you how impossibly challenging it is to control the bodily sensations, nervousness, or sense of dread accompanying your worries, anxieties, and fears. We know that it's difficult not to succumb to the urge to do something to feel better. However, there's no healthy way to discard WAFs; they're part of you, woven into the unique fabric of your history and experiences.

When Control Doesn't Work

Anxiety is universally disliked, and it's natural to want to get rid of it, but simply disliking anxiety doesn't make it a mental health problem or an anxiety disorder. Problems arise when attempts to control anxiety become excessive and inflexible. Such attempts at control lead to ineffective strategies that not only fail to reduce anxiety but also restrict your life and increase your feelings of discontent.

Consider Roger's experience for insight into this cycle.

■ *Roger's Story*

Roger had been battling social anxiety for as long as he could remember. Much of his anxiety and panic centered on his job. He worked hard to prevent his anxiety and panic, but nothing seemed to work. Situations where he had to talk in front of small groups of businesspeople were downright nasty for him: lots of anxiety, sleepless nights beforehand, dread about the possibility of screwing up, making a fool of himself, and being judged. This led Roger to quit his well-paying and interesting job. He ended up taking a back-office job where he didn't have to interact with other people. He earned much less money and felt bored and isolated.

Roger's experience highlights the life-restricting nature of anxiety control efforts. If you've experienced similar struggles, you're not alone. From an early age, most of us are taught that we *should* be able to control our feelings and thoughts. Society also often emphasizes the importance of controlling emotions and thoughts, perpetuating the belief that control is the solution to anxiety.

As you've learned, this approach is fleeting and ultimately ineffective. While control may offer temporary relief, it comes at a high cost. Each moment spent engaging with or avoiding anxiety reinforces the cycle of struggle, leading to increased anticipation and preparation for future WAF attacks.

As Roger discovered, this cycle can consume your life if left unchecked.

> *I cannot and need not control my WAFs. Instead, I can drop the rope to get my life back.*

Anxiety Isn't Like a Hot Stove

As a child you probably avoided touching a red-hot stove because it hurt to touch it. You may have learned this the hard way or by listening to your parents or caregivers warning you about the consequences: "Don't touch _____ because you'll get hurt." Keeping your hand away from hot things kept you from getting burned.

But anxiety doesn't follow the same rules as a hot stove. While avoiding the latter prevents injury, avoiding anxiety only intensifies it. Unlike physical dangers, anxiety thrives on avoidance, growing stronger the more you try to pull away.

Reflect on situations when you've tried to avoid emotional discomfort, akin to pulling away from a hot stove, only to find yourself getting burned anyway.

_____

_____

You've relied on control to navigate external dangers effectively, but applying the same approach to internal pain can backfire. Emotional pain doesn't respond to avoidance like physical danger does.

EXERCISE: Thoughts and Emotions Have No On/Off Switch

Start by getting in a comfortable position. When you're ready, we'd like you to make yourself as happy as you know how to be without thinking about something that makes you happy. Go ahead and try it now. Really work at it.

Could you do it? If you were successful, you most likely recalled a joyful memory or envisioned a pleasant future event. But that's not what we're asking of you. We want you to just flip your super happy switch. Can you do that?

Now, try to make yourself anxious or afraid without focusing on something scary. Just flip the switch. Try hard.

Could you do it? If not convinced about how impossible this is, then try these:

- Force yourself to fall madly and deeply in love with the next person you see.

- Make your left leg completely numb, so if it was pricked by a needle, you wouldn't feel a thing.

We hope this exercise helped you learn that emotions have no on/off switch. It's next to impossible for anyone to feel one way or another just because they want to. Emotions happen as we engage in the world. They're not something we can create out of thin air or stop reliably.

Trying to control unpleasant emotions and thoughts often backfires, triggering more anxiety and fear. Your body operates as an interconnected system, and any attempt to avoid or reduce unpleasant experiences will reverberate throughout the entire system, amplifying your suffering.

The next exercise (adapted from Hayes, Strosahl, and Wilson 2012) will help you experience why struggling with unpleasant feelings and thoughts can make them worse. To begin, find a quiet place where you can sit and get comfortable.

EXERCISE: You're Wired to a Perfect Polygraph and…Zap!

Picture yourself hooked up to the most advanced polygraph machine ever devised, capable of detecting even the faintest hint of anxiety. You can't fool this machine.

Your mission? Stay calm and collected while thinking about a recent anxiety-inducing episode. If successful, you'll walk away with the hefty sum of $100,000.

But there's a twist: any sign of anxiety triggers a lethal shock. The stakes are high, and only complete calmness guarantees survival. So just relax!

Take a moment to jot down what you think would happen in this situation.

Did you manage to claim the prize unscathed, or did anxiety seal your fate? Did anxiety spell disaster?

Every day may feel like a high-stakes game where your life hangs in the balance. You navigate each moment, desperately trying to avoid panic and worry, knowing that one misstep could be fatal.

Then, an invitation to a social gathering arrives. You want to remain calm, but the mere thought of potential awkwardness sends jolts of anxiety through your system—zap, zap, zap. In the end, you bail on your friends, missing out on yet another meaningful experience.

This relentless struggle mirrors being hooked up to the ultimate lie detector: your own nervous system. It's hypersensitive to any hint of anxiety, amplifying your distress as you battle to keep it at bay. With every effort to suppress your fears, the feedback loop intensifies, leaving you feeling increasingly anxious and panicked—zapped once again.

Take Erin, a talented artist whose life is overshadowed by the relentless grip of obsessive-compulsive disorder (OCD).

■ *Erin's Story*

Despite her creative flair and warm personality, Erin is trapped in a world of intrusive thoughts and compulsive behaviors that threaten to suffocate her dreams.

Every day is a battleground as Erin contends with irrational fears and relentless rituals. From meticulously arranging her art supplies to compulsively checking and rechecking her work, OCD dictates every aspect of her life. She's tried many different strategies to resist the fear of making a mistake or causing harm, but it only consumes her thoughts, leaving her paralyzed with anxiety.

Erin's struggle with OCD extends beyond her art studio, infiltrating her relationships and robbing her of joy. She's haunted by a constant need for reassurance and plagued by the fear of others' judgment. Despite her outward success, Erin feels like a prisoner in her own mind, unable to break free from the grip of OCD.

As Erin learned firsthand, trying to suppress thoughts only fuels more unwanted thoughts and emotions. She also learned that trying to control the problem gets in the way of meaningful actions.

To halt this cycle, you'll need to cut off its fuel supply: your unwillingness to accept all aspects of your experience. Your judgmental mind insists you can't be happy with unwanted thoughts and unpleasant emotions. But when you reject this message, you starve the struggle-and-control machine.

Reflect on what struggling has truly brought you—likely little that enriches your life. The good news is that living well doesn't require that you first start feeling and thinking well.

Many people live with immense hardship and yet choose to move forward with meaning and dignity despite pain. How? They don't take the bait. They refuse to spend their valuable time on this earth struggling with their pain. Instead, they acknowledge it without getting ensnared. You're on this path now.

Science and human experience teach us that controlling unwanted psychological and emotional pain only exacerbates it. To get out of this cycle, you'll need to first come to terms with the fact that deliberate control isn't the solution. It's the *problem*. Acceptance, not control, is the key to breaking free from this cycle.

LETTING GO OF THE STRUGGLE FOR CONTROL

Letting go of the struggle for control isn't as hard as it may seem. It begins with you deciding to do so. The hardest part is putting your decision into action.

One of the chief barriers to action is failing to spot places where you have control and places where you don't have much control. To get unstuck and stay that way, you'll need to develop greater ease in the early detection of situations where control is possible in your life. Those places are also where you can make a difference. The next exercise is a preparation for the important work to come.

EXERCISE: What You Can and Cannot Control

Read each statement and then, without much thought, place a circle around those scenarios that you believe you can control. Do not circle anything that you believe is outside your control.

1. What someone else is thinking	9. How others respond to my choices, expressed thoughts, feelings, and actions	17. What other people do
2. The choices I make	10. How I behave with respect to other people	18. Whether I follow certain rules or standards
3. How nervous I get	11. The choices others make	19. Other people liking me
4. How I respond to other people	12. What I do when I get anxious	20. Whether I prepare for tasks and do my best
5. What other people value and care about	13. How often the same thoughts or images come back into my mind	21. What I feel at any point
6. What I say and do in a situation	14. How I respond to my thoughts and feelings (positive or negative)	22. What I do with my precious time on this earth
7. Worries I have from time to time	15. Other people following rules or standards	23. The thoughts I have from time to time
8. The direction I want my life to take	16. Whether I follow through with commitments	24. My values and what I care about

Review any odd-numbered items you circled. These represent situations where you have no control. You may think otherwise, but if you go back and reflect, you'll see that you truly don't have control in any of the odd-numbered scenarios. On the other hand, the even-numbered scenarios demonstrate instances where you do have control. These situations involve your actions and behaviors, offering opportunities to influence outcomes.

Recognize that your mind may falsely suggest you have control when you don't. Struggling to control the uncontrollable leads to increased anxiety and disappointment, empowering WAFs. Instead, when WAFs arise—acknowledge them, pause, and focus on areas where you can exert control over your actions aligned with your values.

THE BIG QUESTION IS ARE YOU WILLING?

Many people have found relief when WAFs arise by observing their bodily sensations, thoughts, and feelings without judgment or resistance. This practice involves simply acknowledging and allowing these experiences to exist without attempting to change them.

It doesn't mean liking what you feel or agreeing with what somebody has done to you. It only means being aware of your anxiety, acknowledging it for what it is—a thought, a feeling, a sensation, a memory, an image—without taking sides or doing anything about it. While this may seem challenging, it offers a new way of relating to anxiety and creates opportunities for new choices and fresh responses. Paradoxically, when you choose to stop struggling and resisting, you're doing something new with your anxiety.

That itself is a big and positive change. You are exercising your ability to choose how you respond: you're taking "response-ability." Responsibility really means that you're able to respond—be response-able—guided by the values in your heart.

Ask yourself who has responsibility for whether or not the WAFs show up. If you think the answer is you, that's just your old conditioning history talking. But now, ask yourself this: *Who can choose and be truly able to respond differently now when WAFs show up?*

We know that dropping the rope in the old tug-of-war is easier said than done. In upcoming chapters, we'll introduce practical exercises to help you embrace this approach and let go of the struggle. You'll cultivate kindness and compassion toward yourself, learning to observe anxiety without being controlled by it.

By prioritizing observation over resistance, you'll enhance your ability to make intentional choices, take action, and lead a fulfilling life. Developing willingness is key to this process.

Willingness Is About Doing

Willingness means making a choice to experience anxiety as it is—a blend of sensations, feelings, thoughts, and images—rejecting the judgment and resistance imposed by your mind. It's akin to taking a leap of faith, diving into life's pool without knowing its temperature or what lies beneath. Unlike wading into the pool and testing the waters cautiously, willingness is unconditional openness to all experiences, regardless of how they may feel.

In fact, if you're willing, stand up (if you can) with arms wide open and stay that way for a bit. While you're standing like this, allow all your experiences to come and be just what they are—make no attempt to change them. Really feel them and let them be. This gesture epitomizes the essence of willingness—a choice to accept and engage with every aspect of life, including anxiety, without fighting it. This itself is a choice; one you can make again and again.

Many people treat anxiety as their worst enemy. But is that true? Must anxiety be your enemy? What if you could learn to develop your willingness muscle? By developing willingness, alongside kindness and compassion for yourself, the need for struggle diminishes. This shift cuts off the fuel supply for anxiety, paving the way for new possibilities aligned with your values and aspirations.

Willingness isn't just a mindset; it's a proactive approach to living authentically. It empowers you to move forward in alignment with your values, irrespective of the fluctuations of the mind and body. It's the catalyst for enacting change and embracing the serenity creed: accepting what cannot be changed while courageously changing what can.

Willingness Makes Growth Possible

It might seem like it would be easier to be willing if you weren't dealing with anxiety, but health isn't about the absence of trauma, pain, or uncomfortable thoughts and feelings. Studies show that willingness to face psychological challenges correlates with better health in all its forms.

Those who embrace their emotional world while pursuing meaningful goals tend to suffer less. Willingness means living a purposeful life with discomfort and difficulties. When you're willing to live such a life, you're on your way out of suffering.

We're not saying this is easy. Setbacks may occur. You may pick up the rope again. When that happens, notice what's going on and make a choice to let it go. Give yourself a few moments to recover. Then decide what you're willing to do next.

Recognizing when you're caught up in old patterns and choosing to let go can lead to growth. By adopting a stance of willingness and making room for anxiety, you can live a fulfilling life.

EXERCISE: Switch On Willingness

Imagine two on/off switches are in front of you. They look like light switches, but one on/off switch is labeled "anxiety," and the other one is labeled "willingness."

The anxiety switch represents how you might have thought about anxiety when you started reading this book. You might have hoped to switch off your anxiety, but this, as you've learned, is a false hope. You can't turn anxiety on or off. You don't have control over it.

Here, we'd like to share an important secret with you. The willingness switch is the one that will make a real difference in your life. Unlike the anxiety switch, you can choose to turn willingness on or off. With willingness, you're not a helpless victim; your actions dictate its state.

You can decide to activate willingness at any time, which may lead to positive changes. It could liberate you from emotional turmoil and empower you to pursue what truly matters to you.

In this metaphor, we're urging you to redirect your focus from what you cannot control to what you can. Have you ever approached anxiety with willingness to experience it? What unfolds might surprise you.

Don't Just Try to Be Willing

"I'll try" is a common initial response when discussing willingness. "Next time I'm anxious, I'll really try to be willing and not do what I usually do." And when things haven't worked out, we hear, "I tried to go to work and face my fear of failure, but I couldn't do it. My anxiety was too much, so I stayed home."

Willingness is not about trying; it's simply about doing or not doing. The following brief exercise is a powerful way to connect with the fact that willingness is an all-or-nothing action. You do it or you don't.

EXERCISE: The Trying Pen

Start by placing a pen in front of you. Now, *try* to pick up the pen. Try as hard as you can.

Did you pick up the pen? But wait, that's not what we asked you to do. We want you to try to pick it up. Try again.

What happens? You either pick up the pen or you don't, right? You realize you can't just try to pick it up. There is no trying.

You may have noticed your hand hovering over the pen when you tried. That's what trying gets you—hovering over your life and not doing what you wish, like trying to lose weight, trying to exercise more, trying to eat healthier foods, trying to do a better job, trying to be more organized, trying to be a more responsive parent or partner, or even trying to be less anxious. Trying leads to paralysis and being stuck.

Trying is really "not doing." This is why we never want you to try anything. Instead, make a choice: if you're completely willing, do it; if you're not willing, don't. Willingness has an on/off switch, not a dial to adjust to be a little bit willing.

Focus on the action, not the results. Even with full willingness, you may not always get what you want. Doing isn't about success or failure; it's about the act itself. For example, you may drop the pen, but you can still pick it up again. Some tasks require repetition and persistence.

When you commit to an action, your mind may flood you with judgmental thoughts, like "See, you tried, but it didn't work out...you're a failure." Let these thoughts pass, and don't let them deter you from what's important. Pick up the pen again. Pick up the pen with the thought of failure.

Remember, willingness is a choice and a commitment to being open to your experiences, even those beyond your control. It will empower you to move forward despite challenges.

Willingness Isn't a Feeling

Many people think of willingness and unwillingness as feelings. But willingness isn't a feeling; it's a choice. We're not asking you to change how you feel about your WAFs; we're asking you to choose to be with them without trying to make them disappear. Why? Because this choice will allow you to do what you care about, regardless of your emotional weather.

If you're willing to make this commitment, sign your name below. If not, take some time to reflect on where you are with your anxiety and what's holding you back from the life you want. Look at the costs of the struggle and the two epitaphs you worked on earlier. Review your Valued Directions Worksheet and Life Compass. You've already taken a bold step by opening this book. You have everything you need to move forward.

The Willingness Commitment

I am willing to think whatever I may think, feel whatever I may feel, and take all of that with me as I use my hands and feet to move myself in directions I want my life to take.

_____   _____
                    Signature   Date

The next exercise will help you build your willingness muscle by adding in the healing qualities of kindness and self-compassion. We recommend that you listen to the audio version available at http://www.newharbinger.com/54476.

EXERCISE: Holding Anxiety Gently

Take a moment to find a quiet, comfortable spot where you won't be interrupted for about five minutes. Sit down, take a few deep breaths in...and out to settle in.

Once you're settled, cup your hands together in your lap, palms facing up. Notice the warmth and openness of your hands, reflecting on the many ways you've used them in your life.

Your hands have been used for work, for love, to touch and be touched, to hold and let go, to create, to express yourself in writing or when speaking with someone, to offer comfort, to heal, and to share kindness. Allow yourself to sink into the goodness contained in your hands.

From this place of kindness, gently allow a small piece of your anxiety to settle into your hands, like a feather floating down. Just let it rest there for a moment, acknowledging its presence without judgment. Just something small—a part of yourself that you might be willing to let rest in your hands.

Notice how it feels to hold this piece of your anxiety with kindness and compassion. Take your time with this experience, breathing deeply and allowing yourself to simply be present. Simply notice, breathe, and sense the warmth and goodness of your hands. There's nothing else to do here. Stay with this experience as long as you wish.

When you're ready, release the anxiety from your hands, like letting go of a butterfly, and take a moment to reflect on what you've learned. Then, when you're ready, open your eyes while reminding yourself that you have the ability to hold your anxiety in a kind way and embrace something new.

If the exercise you just did felt a bit odd, that's okay. Your mind will naturally evaluate your experience—it's what minds do. Instead of blindly rejecting your thoughts and feelings, embrace the opportunity to observe them willingly, with kindness and openness. Each time you consciously respond to your WAFs in this way, you introduce something new, which will lead to significant changes in your life.

LIFE-ENHANCEMENT EXERCISES

You're making significant strides by engaging with the exercises in this workbook. Here's your plan for the week ahead:

- Commit to a daily practice of Holding Anxiety Gently, and observe the effects.

- Continue to work actively with this workbook, completing exercises and reflecting on your progress.

- Use the LIFE Worksheet to identify and track WAFs in your daily life.

- Reflect on your relationship with WAFs. Do you approach them willingly or unwillingly? And with kindness or hostility?

- Practice letting go in situations that are beyond your control.

- Seek support from a trusted individual, sharing your journey and seeking accountability. Ask them to help you notice when you're struggling to control your WAFs.

- Remember, change is ongoing and part of your lifelong journey; it's not a destination. Keep moving forward.

THE TAKE-HOME MESSAGE

You can't control anxiety by avoiding or suppressing it. None of this works. It only buys you more anxiety, frustration, helplessness, and limitation. When your WAFs show up, acknowledge and make room for them instead. Focus on what you can control—your choices and actions—and engage your values and life. Don't forget that.

All the remaining chapters are about fostering your willingness while changing your relationship with your WAFs so that they no longer control you. Willingness is a choice that allows you to maximize control where you have it. This is how you break free from the shackles of anxiety, fears, worry, and other forms of emotional or psychological pain.

Let Go of Struggle for Control and Choose Willingness

Reflections:

- Trying to control my WAFs worsens my anxieties and shrinks my life.

- Making different choices could improve my life.

- There's no trying, only doing. But I must choose to be willing.

Inquiries:

- Am I willing to give up control over what I cannot control to move forward with my life, with or without anxiety?

PART 3

Living Your Life
with or without Anxiety

Take a stand against the habit of chaining yourself to your past and your mistakes. Take a stand against people who have purposefully hurt you time and again. Take a stand against thoughts and opinions seeking to diminish your worth. They shall not move forward with you. You will not allow them to deny you a new beginning. Make a commitment that their part in your life is over and done with, you are far too beautiful and far too strong to be a prisoner of things that do not really matter. Reclaim your life!

—Dodinsky

CHAPTER 10

Becoming an Observer

To be identified with your mind is to be trapped in time: the compulsion to live almost exclusively through memory and anticipation. This creates an endless preoccupation with past and future and an unwillingness to honor and acknowledge the present moment and allow it to be. The compulsion arises because the past gives you an identity and the future holds the promise of salvation, of fulfillment in whatever form. Both are illusions.

—Eckhart Tolle

From the moment of your birth, you've learned to see the world through the veil of thoughts, words, stories, concepts. All of this, including your lived experiences, is part of your learning, or what psychologists call your learning or conditioning history.

Because that's all most of us know, we tend to identify with words and thoughts about ourselves and the world. We then start thinking that what we think is who we are. Tonia referred to "my OCD" as if OCD defined her, while Phil said, "My panic is taking over." It's easy to become so intertwined with thoughts like *I am anxious* or *I am depressed* that we don't realize we're embodying them. Every time we utter "I am," we merge with whatever follows, becoming it. This merging can be unhelpful and quite harmful.

All humans have the capacity to identify with their thoughts and conditioning, but as Eckhart Tolle, Deepak Chopra, and others teach us, this ego self is not who we are. Humans also have the capacity to step back and observe their experiences. You have lots of experience noticing and observing people, places, and objects in your environment. You also know that when you observe an object like a lamp, it doesn't turn you into one. There is a distinction between you and what you observe, sense, and experience, right?

This basic human capacity applies to your inner world too. You can observe your thoughts without buying into them or doing what they say. You can observe your emotions and perhaps use that feedback wisely. The same is true of physical sensations in your body. You can observe the sensation of a toothache, but that doesn't mean you are a toothache. Developing your awareness of the observer part of you is a powerful way to reduce your suffering.

Your thoughts and conditioning can sometimes be helpful. But when they're not, it's important to recognize that there's more to you than your conditioning. Recall that your thoughts and feelings—all of them—are a part of you, but they are not you. The exercises in this chapter will reinforce this important distinction.

YOU ARE MUCH MORE THAN YOUR ANXIETIES AND FEARS

Anxiety and fear are transient emotions, appearing and disappearing like actors on a stage. You, the observer of your life, are distinct from these feelings and thoughts. They may have their time in the spotlight, but you remain the constant observer in the audience of your experience and life. The following imagery exercise will help you get a sense of this observer you.

Imagine the moment of your birth. You and every person on this planet enter the world in the same way. We're born into the world but have no experience of the world. No history. No way to make sense of it. Yet, there you were, with your two eyes looking out onto the world just like every other newborn. In this way, you and everyone else started life much like an empty vessel.

And then quickly, we all start to collect experiences. We taste. We touch. We feel. We begin to speak, talk about our past, ourselves, our future. We're constantly collecting experiences. Some are sweet. Some bitter. Other experiences are mundane. Over time, we notice that our vessel is no longer empty. It will continue to fill for as long as we're alive.

You too have a vessel, containing everything you've lived through and experienced up to this moment in time. And you might spend a lot of time with the stuff you've collected so far. Maybe you identify with it. Maybe you're trying to get rid of some of it, cover things up that you don't like very much, or rearrange things so that your load is easier to carry.

But here, we'd like to ask you a question. What's the one constant that's been with you throughout your life until now? Is it the experiences you've collected? Or, is it that vessel that's pristine you?

That vessel is you—the holder and observer of your life—your safe refuge. That you was there at the moment you came into this world and before the hardship and pain, before the losses and joys, before the trauma, and before anxiety was a problem. It's there always, and with practice you can learn to sense it more clearly and let it help and guide you.

Imagine your favorite piece of music playing. As you listen, your ego self will be evaluating the artist, rhythm, and lyrics. That stuff is a product of your conditioning history. But there's another part of you that's experiencing the music beyond your thoughts and emotions about it. While your ears and brain perceive sound waves and transform them into the notes, it's the silent observer within you—the constant presence—that connects them into the harmonious flow we call music. As Deepak Chopra (2003) affirms, the silent observer part of you bears witness to everything that's going on inside and outside of your mind and body.

You can adopt the silent observer perspective with any experience, even those that trigger anxiety. Notice your heartbeat: who's observing it? It's the silent presence within you, impartially witnessing without judgment. Viewing your experiences from this observer perspective can help you detach from your WAFs. They're just passing waves in the sea of existence. You don't need to fight them or become them. Simply let them come and go, observing from the shore.

So ask yourself if there's enough room inside you to let all of you in—just as you are. If not, what's standing in the way of you experiencing yourself? And if some block shows up, see if you can make space for *that*—not liking or condoning it—just acknowledging that it's there with as much kindness as you can muster and without trying to fix it.

BECOMING AN IMPARTIAL OBSERVER

To truly observe, you must anchor yourself in the present moment, leaving behind thoughts of the past and future. Remember, your life unfolds in the present, and so it needs to be the focal point of your awareness.

Start by tuning in to your body—notice your breath, heartbeat, posture, and any sensations of tension or discomfort. This skill takes practice, which is why we've created several exercises to help you develop it. By mastering these techniques outside of challenging moments, you'll be better equipped to apply them when needed.

The second method to stay present involves monitoring your conscious mind—your thoughts, emotions, and motivations. During WAF episodes, ask yourself essential questions:

- *What emotions am I experiencing aside from anxiety, panic, fear, or tension?*

- *What am I saying to myself, and are these thoughts helpful?*

- *What actions am I inclined to take to avoid discomfort?*

- *What values do I want to prioritize in this moment?*

A helpful mnemonic for staying present is "Watch, look, and listen, or you won't see what you're missing." When negative thoughts arise, don't feed them by engaging with them. If you catch your mind judging, simply observe that thought without self-criticism. Ultimately, a judgment is just another thought. Don't allow it to suck you in. Remember, as the observer, there's no right or wrong—only noticing, experiencing, and learning.

What's It Like to Take the Observer Perspective?

To help you get a feel for the observer self, Pema Chödrön (2001) suggested seeing yourself as the sky and everything else as just the weather. Our Australian colleague Russ Harris (2008) offers a similar weather metaphor that we'd like to share with you here.

Consider your observing self as the vast sky and your thoughts and feelings as clouds drifting across it. You notice that the weather changes all the time. Sometimes the clouds are fluffy and white while at other times they may be dark and stormy. But no matter how bad it gets, the weather is just passing through; it cannot harm the sky.

You are the sky—the expansive, unchanging space within which these thoughts arise and dissolve. This inner sanctuary knows no limits, no boundaries—no beginning, no end. Just as the sky remains unchanged by the presence or absence of clouds, your essential nature remains unaffected by the thoughts and feelings that come and go.

Here, you can discover the power to observe and embrace even the most challenging thoughts and emotions. So, when you notice a thought, see it as simply another cloud passing through your vast sky-like mind.

EXERCISE: **Observing the Mind's Chess Game**

The impartial observer perspective can be illuminated by the game of chess (Hayes, Strosahl, and Wilson 2012). Typically in chess, two players each have a team of pieces and engage in all sorts of moves on the chessboard to win the game. When one player makes a move, the other player takes a piece and makes a counterstrike. In our game, the dark pieces represent your WAFs and everything that might trigger them, and the white pieces represent your counter-strikes to their moves. When the dark knight attacks (with the thought I'm about to lose it), you get on the back of the white knight, ride into battle, and do something to knock the dark knight out: breathe...think of something else...reassure yourself that you can make it.

Looking back at your experience and the work you've done in the previous chapters, ask yourself if this approach has worked. Or does the WAF team always manage to come back and make another move to get you?

In this unique chess game, there's a twist: both teams are one team—you. Every move, thought, and feeling belongs to you, blurring the lines between opponent and strategist. You're both sides, navigating the intricate

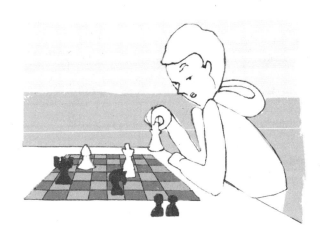

dance between your thoughts, emotions, and actions. It's as if the game were rigged. Your thoughts and feelings play against each other, ensuring that one part of you always loses. In this war against yourself, you simply can't win. You're trapped in a perpetual battle you can't escape, fighting against yourself daily. It feels hopeless.

But let's step back for a moment and look at this situation from a different angle. What if those chess pieces don't represent you? Can you see who else you might be?

What if you're like the chessboard on which the pieces move about? This is an important role. Without the board, there's no game. As the board, you witness all the moves without getting entangled in the outcome.

Imagine the freedom of being the board in the chess game of life. While players are invested in winning, the board doesn't take sides or worry about who wins or loses. It simply provides a space for the game to unfold. Similarly, you can choose to be an impartial observer of your experiences, detached from what arises in your mind and body.

Your thoughts and feelings are like visitors, coming and going, but the board and the sky remain constant. They simply exist, unchanged by the transient experiences that your mind, body, and learning history create.

The human mind creates an illusion that blends feelings, thoughts, actions, and the self into one. When that happens, there's no separation between the you as observer and the you as your learning history. As we suggested, many people identify with their learning history, and that can pull anyone into needless suffering and limitation. This is what needs to change.

EXERCISE: **The Silent Observer Self**

To get a clearer idea of how to separate pieces of your experience from you as observer, consider Ellen's story. Ellen, an office manager, was involved in a serious car accident six months ago. Though she escaped with minor physical injuries, the event left deep emotional scars. She now avoids driving and experiences nightmares, painful memories, and sudden panic attacks. Ellen's work has been affected too. She's on temporary leave and fears losing her job.

Initially, Ellen couldn't differentiate between her fear-related thoughts, feelings, and actions and her observing self, witnessing it all. Instead, they were all crushed together in one upsetting experience. Here's how it looked in a diagram. Notice all the circles are overlapping.

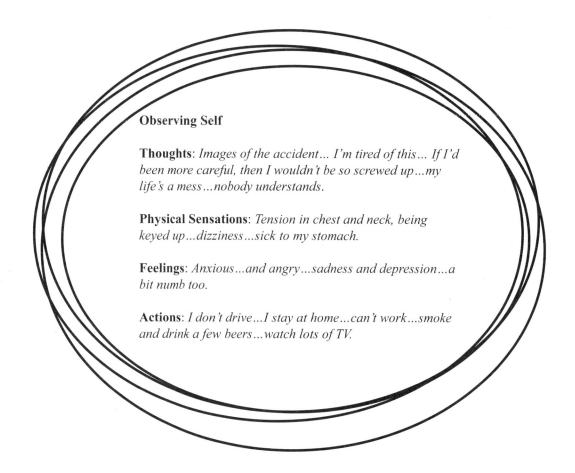

Observing Self

Thoughts: *Images of the accident... I'm tired of this... If I'd been more careful, then I wouldn't be so screwed up...my life's a mess...nobody understands.*

Physical Sensations: *Tension in chest and neck, being keyed up...dizziness...sick to my stomach.*

Feelings: *Anxious...and angry...sadness and depression...a bit numb too.*

Actions: *I don't drive...I stay at home...can't work...smoke and drink a few beers...watch lots of TV.*

To help Ellen distinguish her observing self, her therapist drew a circle on a piece of paper, labeling it "Observing Self (The Silent Observer)." Below this circle, she drew four more circles for thoughts, physical sensations, feelings, and actions.

Her therapist asked Ellen to "bring the chessboard exercise to mind and imagine being the board. This is the place we call the observing self—it's not a real place but a perspective that you can take to look *at* your experiences. It's where you can notice and observe your experiences without having to comment or interfere. Now, from the perspective of that silent observing witness, fill in the other circles."

Here's what the exercise looked like once Ellen completed it. As you can see, the four circles are no longer overlapping. Thoughts, physical sensations, feelings, and actions are now distinct yet connected to and in touch with her observing self.

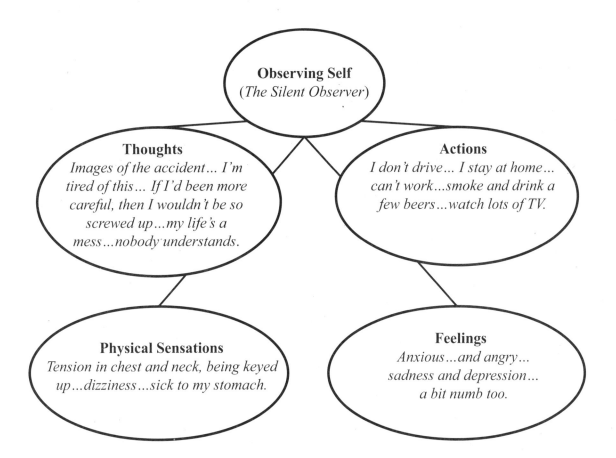

Right now, we'd like you to engage in this same exercise using a recent WAF experience you've had. Download the Silent Observer Self Worksheet from http://www.newharbinger .com/54476. Then, gather your recent LIFE Worksheets and select one that encapsulates a challenging situation for you. Take a moment to review what you wrote down.

When you're ready, focus on the gentle rhythm of your breath, feeling it rise and fall in your chest and belly. Simply observe it for a few moments until you feel centered. Now, visualize the WAF episode from your LIFE Worksheet. From the viewpoint of your silent observing self, dissect each aspect of the experience. Distinguish your thoughts, feelings, physical sensations, and actions. Then, as Ellen did, record your observations on your Silent Observer Self Worksheet.

There's one more important insight that can be gleaned from the exercise you just did. Your behavior is separate from your thoughts and feelings. You can be awash with anxious thoughts and feelings and still choose to act in ways that are meaningful. Your thoughts and feelings do not create actions. You do!

The key takeaway here is the power of awareness: you can observe all your experiences and still choose your actions. One set of actions is to act on your anxiety by trying to stuff or bury it. Another is to do what your history and mind tell you to do, which is likely to avoid or escape from painful aspects of your history. And here's a third one: you can observe the discomfort arising from your mind and body with compassion, kindness, gentle curiosity, and openness, viewing it from the standpoint of you as the silent observer. When you do that, you avoid taking sides or passing judgment, leaving space for actions that could enrich your life. Whenever you forget that your behavior is a choice, you're unlikely to exercise choice. You'll let your old habitual history take over, where your thoughts and feelings drive what you do.

Practice developing your silent observing skills with the WAF experiences recorded in your LIFE Worksheets. Start with less challenging episodes and commit to at least one silent observer practice daily. Simply notice and watch your thoughts and feelings, then place each in its own bubble with gentle kindness and compassion. Notice the difference between you (the silent observer) and your thoughts, sensations, feelings, and actions. This approach empowers you to choose your actions consciously rather than be driven by inner turmoil.

WHO ARE YOU, REALLY?

When asked "Who are you?" many people respond with their name or their roles in life: mother, coach, doctor, construction worker, lawyer, receptionist, artist. But is this who you really are—your body? Your roles? Your name?

Deep down, we all intuitively sense there's a part of us that remains unchanged despite changing circumstances. For instance, there was a time when you called yourself a first grader, and now you call yourself something else, but there was a you that was there back in first grade and that's still here with you now. Remember you were there before you had words to describe you!

Persisting with the question "Who are you?" often elicits responses like "I'm anxious," "I'm a good person," or "I'm terrible at math." Try it yourself: "I am _____." Fill in the blank with whatever shows up.

These self-descriptions often evolve into elaborate narratives about your identity. While storytelling is natural, it's crucial to remember that such narratives are just that—stories, products of the mind. Stories may contain facts and truths about your lived experiences, and you should acknowledge and honor them. But clinging to a narrative that no longer serves you can, and often will, hinder your growth.

For instance, you may believe that you've always been an anxious person. Your mind may offer you at least ten reasons why you've become such a person and then tell you that you can't go out because you're an anxious person. If you buy into this story, you won't go out and may find your life shrinking around you. In fact, such stories can become utterly self-defeating life traps if you really believe them *and* do as they say.

To interrupt this process, it's crucial to discern between acknowledging your experiences and buying into unhelpful narratives that feed suffering and shrink your life. With any story or narrative your mind creates, you can always pause and then ask, *Is this story helpful, guiding me forward into the life I desire?*

At this point, you may ask, "If I'm not my body or my thoughts, feelings, actions, or words about myself, then who am I?" This is an important question. Let's explore this question without falling back on familiar narratives.

EXERCISE: "Who Am I (Beyond My WAFs)?"

Due to years of dealing with your WAFs, you may have fixated on what seems to be wrong with you, losing sight of other important aspects of yourself and your life. In this exercise, we invite you to reflect on key facets of yourself and your life unrelated to your WAFs. Describe yourself and your preferences, completing each line below. If you struggle with any, recall a time before your WAFs were a major problem in your life and then complete the item.

I am _____ / _____ / _____ / _____ / _____.

I am a person who _____.

I am not someone who _____.

I really like _____.

I do not like _____.

My most important relationship is _____.

How else would you describe yourself? _____

_____

_____

_____

_____

We know that words can never fully capture who we are. Our essence transcends language—it's an unlimited and unbounded refuge. The exercises in this chapter aim to help you experience this profoundly safe aspect of yourself, beyond definitions and words and apart from everything you've accumulated in your vessel up until now.

To guide you in experiencing your inner sanctuary, untouched by stories or descriptions, let's begin with an exercise inspired by Roberto Assagioli (1973) and adapted by Hayes, Strosahl, and Wilson (2012). This exercise invites you to use your imagination to reach a place where you can transcend your stories. You can listen to and download it at http://www.newharbinger.com/54476.

EXERCISE: The Constant Observer

Close your eyes, get settled in your chair, and simply follow the instructions. If you ever find your mind wandering, just gently come back to the sound of the voice.

Before we start, take a couple of gentle breaths—in...and out...in...and out. As you're doing so, notice the sound and feel of your own breath. Now turn your attention to being just where you are, here in this room sitting in a chair.

Now imagine you're watching yourself in a mirror. The eyes looking back at you now are the very same eyes that were also there on your first day of school. Can you still remember that day? What did you see with your eyes then? And what was happening inside of you that day? Do you notice any emotions you were having... Any thoughts? Now I want you to notice that, as you noticed these things, there was a part of you noticing them. A part of you noticed those sensations...those sounds...thoughts...and feelings. And that part of you we will call the "observer you." There is a person in here, behind those eyes, who is aware of what I am saying right now. And it is the same person you've been all your life. In some deep sense, this observer you is that you, which you call "you."

Now I want you to remember the day you met your first girlfriend or boyfriend, or if your memory of that event is too faint, then remember the day you met your current partner... The eyes looking back at you from the mirror are the very same eyes that were there with you then, noticing everything that was happening... Remember all the things that were happening then... Remember the sights...the sounds...the smells...your feelings...your thoughts...and as you do, see if you can notice that you were there then, noticing what you were noticing. See if you can catch the person behind your eyes who saw, heard, smelled, felt, and had thoughts... You were there then, and you are here now... We're just asking you to notice the experience of being aware and to check and see if, in some deep sense, the you who is here now was also there then... The person aware of what you are aware of now is here now, and that person was also there then.

Behind those eyes you see in the mirror now is the same you who was with you when you were a kid on vacation with your family, later in high school, in college, and still later on the job... It's also the same you who is with you today when you leave the house in the morning, when you check your cell phone, go shopping, and when you're having dinner together with friends...

What is important here is this: during all these moments you saw different things, had different thoughts, and experienced different feelings. Your looks have changed a lot over time as well. But one thing hasn't changed: it has always been the same pair of eyes that during all these different experiences looked *at* these experiences and watched everything. The observer behind your eyes was there then, and it is here now—and that observer was the same then as it is now... Again, we're asking you not to believe this; just see if you notice this basic continuity—in some deep sense at the level of experience, not at the level of belief. This observer has always been the same. You have been you your whole life.

Your roles are constantly changing too. Sometimes you're a friend, a parent, a colleague, a business partner, a romantic partner. But no matter what role you happen to be playing at any given time, there is a you there behind your eyes who is not changing but simply observing how you move through life playing out all those different roles.

Now finally, let's look at your emotions. Notice how your emotions are constantly changing. Sometimes you feel joyful, sometimes you feel sad. At other times, you feel tense...and then comes boredom...excitement...relaxation. And yes, while these emotions come and go, notice that in some real sense the you who is registering all these changing emotions does not change... The same is true for your thoughts. They come and go, seemingly out of nowhere, and then go back there again... Sometimes you think about others, sometimes you think about yourself. Sometimes your thoughts make sense to you, and sometimes they don't.

So, as a matter of experience, not of belief, can you sense that you're not just your body... your roles...your emotions...your thoughts? All of these are the content of your life, while you are the arena...the place...the space in which they unfold... Notice that the worries, anxieties, and fears you've been struggling with and trying to change are not you. No matter how long this war goes, *you* will be there, unchanged and safe... See if you can take advantage of this connection to let go of your worries, anxieties, and fears just a little bit, secure in the knowledge that you have been you through it all, and that you need not be so invested in your emotional weather as a measure of your life... Instead, just notice the experiences in all the areas of your life that show up, and as you do, notice that *you* are still here, being aware of what you are aware of... *That* does not change.

Take a moment longer and just stay with this silent, unchanging, constant witness... Then when you're ready, picture yourself sitting on your chair in your room. And after a moment or two, come back to your room and open your eyes.

The Constant Observer exercise will help you adopt the observer perspective across various aspects of your life while offering a glimpse into the safe sanctuary within you. We recommend listening to this exercise several times weekly in the coming weeks to familiarize yourself with the silent witnessing observer—your authentic self and steadfast ally amidst all the fluctuations of the mind and body.

FINDING YOUR TRUE SELF

Becoming a skilled observer offers a valuable perspective and experience for anyone struggling with WAFs and other forms of emotional or psychological pain. To understand its significance, consider the following list of statements. Reflect on your internal response as you read the first four statements, then continue by completing the last four statements with troubling self-descriptions that your mind frequently presents to you:

- I am an anxious person.

- I am too shy.

- I am not good enough.

- I am never going to make it.

- I am _____.

- I am _____.

- I am _____.

- I am not _____.

Did you notice how quickly your mind started to work on these statements, perhaps agreeing or disagreeing with them, rephrasing or qualifying them, making them stronger, toning them down, and so on? You're accustomed to being ensnared by such self-descriptions, spending considerable time and energy struggling with and reacting to them—the familiar tug-of-war scenario. But our mind just makes up all these *I am this* or *that* statements. It's an unhelpful illusion to think that you are what you think and feel. The only constant truth and reality is *I Am*—period!

This is not just some abstract philosophical idea but a very practical and helpful skill to learn. After engaging in the tug-of-war exercise, many people ask, "How do I let go of the rope in daily life? How do I stop engaging when my mind bombards me with evaluative 'I am this or that' and 'I'm-not-good-enough' statements?" Here's what you do.

You affirm that you are neither this nor that. You are not the labels and stories your mind creates. Instead, you acknowledge that *I Am*. Responding to the question *Who am I really?* with a simple, disarming *I Am* enables you to release all those evaluative self-statements your mind incessantly creates. It's the simplest and most effective way to drop the rope—anytime. No more debates, explanations, or justifications—simply, *I Am that I Am!*

Simply think or say *I Am* silently to yourself whenever your mind is trying to lure you into a discussion of who or what you are.

Ancient Wisdom Practice for Modern Minds

The "I Am" meditation is a short form of a very old mantra "I Am that I Am." It transcends boundaries and resonates across ancient wisdom traditions, including mentions in the Old Testament and Sanskrit scriptures (Dyer 2012). Mantras have held the key to a profound inner journey across different cultures for centuries. Rooted in ancient tradition, they are specific sounds with well documented mental and physical healing and other beneficial properties.

The following exercise is designed to teach you to drop all those unhelpful evaluative statements about yourself in your daily life. Every time you practice, you begin to go beyond the turbulent waves of your thoughts and feelings by letting go of all that old negative self-talk and simply affirming "I…Am."

EXERCISE: "I Am" Meditation

Find a comfortable position to sit… Allow your eyes to close gently… Take a deep breath in…and slowly exhale, letting go of any tension… Continue to breathe deeply, allowing each breath to bring you into a deeper state of calm and relaxation.

As your breath flows gently in and out, allow your mind to quiet down, releasing any thoughts that may arise… If your mind wanders, let it be and do what it does. Do not control or focus on anything. Simply allow your experience to be what is without trying to change anything.

Now, silently begin to repeat the words "I…Am." With each inhale, silently say "I," and with each exhale, say "Am." Feel the power of these words resonate within you. "I…Am."

As you continue to breathe and repeat these words silently in your mind, allow yourself to connect with the essence of who you are. Feel a sense of peace and presence washing over you. "I…Am."

With each breath, affirm your existence and your unique presence in this world. "I…Am." There is no need to add anything to this statement. "I Am" is enough. It is a declaration of your being, of your existence, of your presence in this moment. "I…Am."

Feel the energy of "I…Am" filling your body. Let it expand and radiate throughout your entire being. Feel it in your heart, your mind, your soul. "I…Am."

As you continue to repeat these words, allow any feelings of doubt or unworthiness to dissolve. Trust that you are enough just as you are. "I…Am."

Take a few more minutes just feeling the peace and stillness within you. "I…Am."

When you're ready, gently bring your awareness back to the room… Then slowly open your eyes. Carry the essence of "I Am" with you throughout your day, knowing and trusting that you are enough just as you are.

We suggest practicing the "I Am" meditation at least once a day, preferably twice a day. With the suggested approximate timing, the entire practice will only take about eight to nine minutes. Regularly practicing the "I Am" meditation will prove to be a valuable step on your journey toward learning to let go of your old unhelpful negative self-talk.

In addition, if you want to "turbo-charge" your progress toward quieting your mind more generally and experiencing your true inner self—your transcendent self—we recommend you learn transcendental meditation (TM). TM is the meditation technique with the most extensive research base attesting to its beneficial effects on psychological well-being and physical health (Sedlmeier et al. 2012). Our recommendation to learn TM is based not only on this impressive research record but also on our own personal experience with having practiced TM for many years.

TM is a simple, effortless, and natural way of transcending (literally "going beyond") the turbulent waves of your thoughts and feelings. You regularly dive into the serene depths of pure consciousness that reside within you—your true Self. This practice teaches you to allow all thoughts and feelings to be there. You also learn to let go of any expectations or attempts to control the experience including your anxiety. This is why practicing TM is so helpful when you've been struggling with anxiety (Orme-Johnson and Barnes 2014).

The TM technique doesn't take long to learn and is easy to practice. You typically practice twice a day for about twenty minutes. Meditations like TM have been passed down for thousands of years only orally and directly from an expert teacher to a student desiring to learn. This is still the case today. A mantra most suitable for you is personally selected by a qualified TM teacher and taught in a very specific way individually and in a private session by the teacher. You can find more information and a qualified teacher at http://www.tm.org (see also Roth 2022).

LIFE-ENHANCEMENT EXERCISES

Consider the activities listed below as essential self-care practices, tailored to your needs. Put them on your to-do list each day. Set an intention to practice the exercises. Choose any activity that resonates with you and commit to doing it wholeheartedly.

Also be realistic in your commitments, aiming for what you can genuinely accomplish. For instance, if twice-daily "I Am" meditation feels overwhelming, commit to once daily. Quality over quantity matters—better to fulfill realistic goals consistently than to overcommit and not follow through. If you find yourself unable to commit, pause and reflect on potential barriers. Maybe slowing down and revisiting earlier exercises are necessary before you move on. Your journey is unique—prioritize your well-being at your own pace.

We understand that change can feel scary. But if you desire a new outcome, you must embrace fresh approaches and do something new. This requires patience and effort, but the rewards are worth it. Stay committed to doing the work—it will yield results. Your own experiences will validate this truth over time.

- Practice the "I Am" meditation at least once, preferably twice a day for ten minutes. If possible, use the audio or be sure to read the instructions before you start your meditation.

- Practice being a mindful silent observer (the chessboard or vessel) during everyday activities at home and elsewhere—this can actually be very funny.

- Practice taking the perspective of the silent observer within you when something upsets or scares you. Notice the distinction between you and your thoughts, feelings, physical sensations, and behaviors.

- Practice being more mindful in your daily life.

- Take stock and notice what your experience is telling you. Even noticing your mind wandering is a good sign—a sign that you're becoming more skillful at observing your experience and not buying everything your mind sells you.

- Use the exercise What I Gave Up for Anxiety (in chapter 7) to explore what you may still be giving up for anxiety this week.

THE TAKE-HOME MESSAGE

Your thoughts, feelings, and actions are not your true self. Your true self is a witnessing observer of all your experiences. By adopting this perspective of you as your observing self, you gain the space needed to focus on creating the life you desire. Becoming a more accepting and compassionate observer of your experiences cultivates flexibility and softness with internal sources of pain and difficulty while also fostering kindness toward yourself and others. This undermines the power of familiar patterns that keep you stuck and suffering, and paves the way for growth and change.

Mastering Perspective Taking: Becoming the Silent Observer

Reflections:

- Recognizing my thoughts, feelings, and actions as distinct from my true self is a courageous leap forward. I am not my WAFs; I am the one who notices them. This silent observing self is my steadfast ally amidst all fluctuations of the mind.

- Embracing the role of a compassionate observer allows for easier self-acceptance and gentler navigation through life's challenges.

Inquiries:

- Am I willing to witness my flaws, hurts, and vulnerabilities from a detached standpoint, rather than engaging with them as an active participant?

- Will I commit to learning to separate my core self from my thoughts, feelings, physical sensations, and behaviors, through consistent I Am meditation, paving the way for personal growth to reclaim control over my life?

CHAPTER 11

Mindful Acceptance

Water is fluid, soft, and yielding. But water will wear away rock, which is rigid and cannot yield. As a rule, whatever is fluid, soft, and yielding will overcome whatever is rigid and hard.

—Lao Tzu

Take a moment and allow yourself to sit with the opening quote of this chapter, for it contains a profound truth that could change your life. As Lao Tzu teaches us, strength lies in softness. Let this powerful message sink in, for everything you're about to learn rests on this insight.

Anxiety and fear often lead us to harden. We then tend to meet this hardness with more hardness, and this only increases our suffering and creates more limitation. You likely know this yourself. So what can you do instead?

Simply, you need to learn to soften when you're inclined to stiffen, expand when you'd rather contract, to lean into life and open when your impulse is to turn away and close. Above all, you learn to nurture your capacity for gentleness, kindness, and compassion in relation to your mind, your body, and the world. These supple, adaptable, and healing qualities are powerful antidotes to human suffering and can be summed up in two words: mindful acceptance.

Mindful acceptance is a stance toward life: observing struggle without judgment, feeling pain without allowing yourself to be consumed by it, and honoring your wounds without embodying them. It's not a feeling or a mindset. It doesn't come from crystals or epiphanies either.

Instead, it's an ongoing practice of choosing to be willing to experience your self and the contents of your vessel just as they are, and then responding to them with the same quality you would share with a loved one who's hurting (Brach 2004). Mindful acceptance is a skill that will offer you genuine freedom from suffering but also requires practice and effort to master.

Before starting that journey, we'd like you to do this exercise.

EXERCISE: Visualizing the Soft-Rock WAF Shuffle

This exercise will help you connect with what a softer response can offer you in relation to your WAFs. Find a quiet and comfortable place. Then allow yourself a moment to think about your WAFs. Let all the words that come to mind pour forth, unedited. In the space below, write all of them down as quickly as they come to you.

Here's how Matt, who had a long history of suffering with panic, described his WAFs: My WAFs are *nasty, crippling, intense, overwhelming, gripping, painful, a burden, a wall, a knife, screwed up, exhausting, shameful, embarrassing.*

Now it's your turn. *My WAFs are* _____

Once you've poured out your thoughts, immerse yourself in the negative energy, the hardness of the words your mind used to describe your WAFs. Take a moment to truly feel it.

Now, transition gently to the first word from the list below. Absorb it slowly, closing your eyes and reflecting on its essence. Imagine embodying the action or feeling implied by the word when your WAFs show up. Allow each subsequent word in the list to wash over you, connecting with its inherent quality. Imagine breathing in each word and allowing it to fill your mind and body fully. This is the softer response we're after.

I will meet my hard WAFs with these qualities:

Softness · Gentleness · Kindness · Openness · Compassion

Love · Patience · Humor · Caring · Curiosity

We'd like you to repeat this exercise now by shuttling back and forth between the *hard* words you came up with about your WAFs and each *softer* response option below. Continue this back and forth. Imagine yourself meeting your *hard* WAFs with each *softer* response. Give yourself at least one minute with each new response option.

After completing this brief exercise, did you notice any shifts? Did the quality of your thoughts about your WAFs change, even just a little bit, as you cycled back and forth through each softer response option? This may be hard to detect. Here's another way to think about it: after doing the exercise, would you describe your WAFs using the same words as before? Or, even if you chose to use the same words, do you really need to buy into them and do what they say?

Don't worry if you didn't notice anything dramatic here. The intent of the exercise is to reveal, even if only in a small way, what the softness of mindful acceptance can offer you. It has the power to erode the hardness of your WAFs and diminish the urge to constantly engage with them. However, mastering mindful acceptance requires practice just like any skill. Remember, softness will wear away rock—the hardness that underlies your tendency to struggle, to fight, and to pick up the rope in a tug-of-war with anxiety.

You possess the ability to choose this softer, more skillful approach. With time and practice, you'll find that mindful acceptance goes beyond anxiety—it's applicable to all aspects of life. Mastering this skill set will enrich your life in countless ways.

UNLOCKING THE POWER OF ACCEPTANCE

Many people have told themselves at some point, *I just need to accept my anxiety.* In fact, we hear it quite a bit. You may have told yourself that too. Still, acceptance is poorly understood, and many people don't know what it really means.

Acceptance is not merely passive acquiescence; it's not about succumbing to your pain, giving up, or resigning yourself to defeat. Also, acceptance is not about doing nothing in the face of circumstances where you have control. So, we're not asking you to accept a bad situation if there's something you can do to change it.

Unfortunately, misconceptions about acceptance tether many people to a cycle of stagnation and self-deprecation. They give up and stop making efforts to change. By viewing acceptance through a lens of passivity, you relinquish control by letting your WAFs (something you cannot control) dictate your actions (something you can control).

Authentic acceptance, by contrast, is an active process. As such, you're making a choice to be open to what's happening anyway, just as it is, and about which you have no control—think your thoughts, feelings, physical sensations, or the behavior and reactions of other people in your life. It's about acknowledging your experiences without judgment or resistance, empowering you to navigate life's challenges with resilience and clarity.

Rather than succumbing to defeat, genuine acceptance liberates you from the shackles of struggle and self-doubt, guiding you toward growth and self-empowerment. Embracing acceptance is not a concession—it's a bold declaration of your capacity to transcend adversity and cultivate inner strength.

As you work to cultivate genuine acceptance, brace yourself for loud protest and resistance from your mind. Your mind likely has ingrained the belief that anxiety is your enemy, one that's entwined with every aspiration and facet of your life. It wants to convince you that your anxious distress is a barrier standing between you and your life, so you need to do something about it.

This might leave you feeling trapped between two unfavorable options: passively succumbing to emotional pain and doing nothing or fervently battling against it, risking the erosion of significant aspects of your life. The first is passive acceptance and the second is flat-out nonacceptance. Both are unhelpful. You're lived experience tells you as much.

However, a transformative third option—mindful acceptance—is worth exploring. Mindful acceptance presents a promising alternative, offering potential pathways to growth and well-being. Be forewarned: the practice itself may feel counterintuitive, and it should. Mindful acceptance asks you to do the opposite of what you tend to do when emotional discomfort shows up.

The next exercise will help you get a sense of what we mean by doing the opposite and how it can be liberating.

EXERCISE: Chinese Finger Trap

A Chinese finger trap is a novelty toy traditionally made of woven straw or bamboo, though modern versions may use other materials like plastic. It typically consists of a hollow tube, approximately five inches in length and half an inch in width, with openings at both ends. Perhaps you can find one at a novelty or party store and use it as you follow along. If you don't have one, visualize the experience.

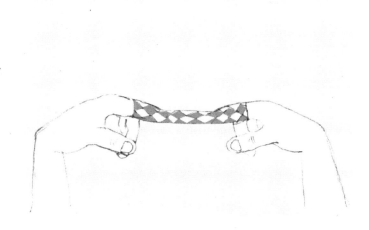

To use the finger trap, you insert an index finger from each hand into the opposite ends of the tube. You push them in as far as you can and then try to pull them out. Initially, this seems straightforward, but the design of the trap includes an inward-facing weave pattern that constricts when tension is applied, effectively trapping your fingers inside.

Despite its simplicity, the Chinese finger trap presents a perplexing challenge: the more you struggle to pull your fingers out, the tighter the trap becomes. This creates a counterintuitive experience, where attempting to escape the trap only exacerbates the situation, leading to a sense of entrapment. That's exactly how the WAF trap works.

The finger trap illustrates how our instinctive responses to emotional pain often keep us stuck and create even bigger problems. Similarly, attempting to avoid anxiety and fear only intensifies these feelings, trapping you in a cycle of discomfort and adversity. Your experience with anxiety tells you that this struggle has only brought you more discomfort and life problems. You're *trapped*!

However, there's a counterintuitive solution supported by our research: instead of pulling away, you do the opposite—you push inward. If you did this with a finger trap, you'd notice that pushing in creates space, offering flexibility and relief. This is what acceptance offers.

Acceptance is doing something counterintuitive. As you practice leaning into pain and anxiety rather than pulling away, you'll be learning to stay with your experience. You acknowledge the discomfort and make room for it, allowing it to be, without doing anything about it and without trying to make it go away. This will give you room to live your life.

THE FOUR QUALITIES OF MINDFUL ACCEPTANCE

Mindfulness and acceptance are difficult concepts to pin down for many people, including us. Some associate mindful acceptance with religious practices like Buddhism; yet, the practice of mindful acceptance actually transcends religious boundaries. That said, there's some consensus about four qualities that go into mindful acceptance.

Jon Kabat-Zinn (1994), a noted mindfulness scholar and therapist, packs the essential qualities of mindfulness into the following definition: "paying attention in a particular way: on purpose, in the present moment, and nonjudgmentally" (p. 4). Let's unpack each part before we go forward with the practice.

Paying Attention

Navigating the present moment is a daunting task, as you contend with distractions from both external sources and your internal thoughts and sensations. Both sources can pull you out of the present in a flash. If you've suffered a past trauma or relive painful memories, then you know this pull and how it can trap you in cycles of rumination and distress.

On top of that, your critical judgmental mind will often hijack your attention, keeping you preoccupied with past regrets, old wounds, and future worries. This mental chatter distracts you from the present moment and will often distort it. Frank's experience with panic attacks illustrates how the mind can distort benign physical sensations.

Often, when Frank was in the throes of a panic attack, he would focus on his heart and feel it beating rapidly. His mind told him, *This is really bad…you're dying…you're going lose it and humiliate yourself.* Until Frank started learning mindful acceptance, he saw no difference between what his mind told him and his actual experience of a fast-beating heart. So, he reacted to physical sensations and his life based on ingrained unhelpful habits, and this further distanced him from the present and his desired path.

Mastering the art of mindful attention—fully engaging with the present moment without defense—can break these patterns of distraction and mental distortion. By embracing the present, you forge a deeper connection with yourself and your surroundings, fostering vitality and growth. Without attentive awareness, there's no way to learn and grow.

So, as you learn to pay attention, you're making a choice to notice what's happening just as it is. This noticing is the opposite of looking away or getting tangled up in your mind's commentary about you and your lived experiences. Instead, you notice any mental chatter as more thinking.

On Purpose

To pay attention, you must consciously choose to do it, and do it again and again, over and over throughout your day and your life. This alone can be difficult to do. Yet, by doing so, you break from old patterns and take control, observing with gentle curiosity the unfolding of each moment. This deliberate shift interrupts the cycle of unproductive strategies that have kept you stuck. Rather than withdrawing, you intentionally lean into your experiences.

At times, you may regress into familiar automatic patterns. The key is recognizing these moments, recommitting to mindful action, and refocusing on the present as things are, not as how your mind says they are. Instead of berating yourself for "failing," celebrate your awareness of these old habits. You might just say, *There's my old history again*. Acknowledge all of it without judgment, express gratitude for the reminder, and gently redirect your attention to what truly matters in the moment.

In the Present Moment

The human mind tends to wander, pulling each of us away from the present moment more often than we realize. Whether it's showering while mentally planning your day or driving on autopilot, these experiences illustrate how easily you can lose touch with the present.

Being lost in thought means missing out on the richness of the present—the only tangible reality. Studies also show that our happiness tanks the more we allow our minds to wander away from the present. Mindful acceptance serves as a compass, guiding you back to the here and now, enabling a deeper connection with your surroundings and yourself.

This skill not only provides clarity and perspective but also anchors you in the here and now. Given that life unfolds moment by moment, being present is essential for fully experiencing and engaging with life.

Nonjudgmentally

Learning to let go of judgment is perhaps the most challenging aspect of mindful acceptance, and it's a process that unfolds gradually. The challenge lies in the human tendency to dwell in our thoughts, constantly interpreting and evaluating our experiences.

We all have this tendency and can apply it to nearly everything—ourselves, others, and situations—often triggering a chain reaction of escalating distress. The judgmental mind wrenches you away from the present, plunging you into a cycle of habitual reactions. Before you know it, you're stuck holding the rope, ensnared in a struggle with yourself, trapped in familiar patterns of seeking comfort and safety.

You know the ways you judge situations, other people, and your own thoughts, feelings and behaviors: *This is horrible! What an idiot! How could I do that?! I can't take this anymore! Why can't I be normal?* or *Here I go again.* These judgments fuel the struggle with your WAFs, perpetuating a cycle of negativity and inner turmoil. None of it is helpful to you.

Positive judgments can be just as harmful: *I need...I want...I should have...or I deserve...* These thoughts stem from a belief that something is lacking or must be obtained. When you cling to these thoughts, especially when they arise automatically and intensely, you lose sight of what truly matters, falling into a cycle of struggle and self-blame.

The issue lies in your attachment to these judgments—taking them too seriously. While it's impossible to stop your mind from producing judgments, the key is to observe them without acting on them and doing as they say, especially when they're unhelpful.

Every judgment creates a distorted reality, leading you to chase after elusive qualities like peace of mind or happiness, as if they were tangible possessions. Judgment also fuels the struggle to remove unpleasantness. But happiness, like all emotions, fluctuates over time—it cannot be grasped and held like a physical object.

Pause for a moment and reflect on your own experience. Can happiness be obtained and kept like a can of soda, or does it ebb and flow like other thoughts and emotions? When you act on the belief that you can possess certain emotions and get rid of others, you'll invite misery.

Pulling It Together

Putting acceptance into action is a potent antidote to the suffering driven by WAFs. Why? Because acceptance means that you're willing and open to experiences as they arise and over which you have no control and you welcome them with qualities of compassion, kindness, and even some playfulness. When combined with mindful attention, free from judgment and anchored in the present moment, these softer qualities dissolve the need to struggle, granting you the freedom to pursue what truly matters.

Initially, embodying nonjudgmental qualities might pose a challenge, particularly in the face of adversity. Yet, acknowledging judgments as mere products of the mind allows you to label them as

The Mindfulness & Acceptance Workbook for Anxiety

"thinking," gradually reducing their impact over time. Remember, you have a choice in this matter, and your mind will give you ample opportunities for practice.

Facing discomfort with mindful acceptance can be challenging, as our human instinct is often to flee from what we dislike. However, mindful acceptance doesn't require us to enjoy unpleasant feelings; it simply involves acknowledging them without resistance, avoidance, or escape. By ceasing the struggle against these feelings, you free up energy to shape the life you desire.

As you journey through this process, you'll realize that your WAFs are merely transient phenomena, coming and going on their own like the weather. With practice, you'll learn to observe judgments and urges with gentle curiosity and kindness.

Despite the challenges, the choice to embrace mindful acceptance is yours. By offering kindness and gentle attention to your inner experiences, you befriend yourself, affirming and welcoming all facets of your emotional landscape. This is one of the kindest things you can do for yourself. It will empower you to navigate life's complexities with grace and resilience.

MINDFUL ACCEPTANCE PRACTICE

Mindfulness exercises teach us that we can't control what enters our minds or what we feel. We can only choose what to pay attention to, how we pay attention, and how we respond. The exercise below will help you do just that. It ought to take about fifteen minutes.

In this exercise, we again focus on the breath—a constant, shifting element like your thoughts and feelings. This exercise will help you develop the skill of paying attention to your breathing while allowing thoughts, feelings, or physical sensations to come and go without getting tangled up in them. If you pay attention with a quality of openness and compassion, you'll see that all of this activity does change from moment to moment without effort on your part. With time, you'll also realize that no matter how bad an internal experience seems, it neither lasts forever nor can it do you any harm.

We'd like you to keep in mind that this exercise isn't about making you feel different, better, relaxed, or calm. This may happen or it may not. The idea is to bring a kindhearted awareness to *any* sensations that show up, including any thoughts or worries that come into your mind. It's about learning to stay with your WAFs with loving-kindness toward yourself, bringing as much warmth and compassion into the situation as you can. This is a concrete way of learning that anxiety isn't the enemy.

With practice, you'll eventually be able to apply this skill of mindful acceptance in your life, anytime or anyplace. There's no right or wrong way to practice. The important thing is that you commit to doing these exercises on the path of becoming a more mindful observer and full participant in your life.

Find a quiet, comfortable space—your healing space—and listen to the guided audio available on the workbook website. After some time, you might choose to practice without guidance. You can always return to the audio recording for support.

EXERCISE: Acceptance of Thoughts and Feelings

Get in a comfortable position in your chair. Sit upright with your feet flat on the floor, your arms and legs uncrossed, and your hands resting in your lap (palms up or down, whichever is more comfortable). Allow your eyes to close gently.

Take a few moments to get in touch with the movement of your breath and the sensations in your body. As you do that, slowly bring your attention to the gentle rising and falling of your breath in your chest and belly. Like ocean waves coming in and out, your breath is always there. Notice its rhythm...the changing patterns of sensations...the temperature of the air as it passes in and out of your nose...the movement in your chest and belly. Take a few moments to feel the physical sensations of the breath moving in...and out.

There's no need to control your breathing. Simply let the breath breathe itself. As best you can, bring an attitude of generous allowing and gentle acceptance to your experience, just as it is.

Sooner or later your mind will wander away from the breath to other concerns, thoughts, worries, images, bodily sensations, planning, or daydreams, or it may just drift along. This is what minds do much of the time. When you notice your mind has wandered, just acknowledge that awareness of your experience. Then, gently, and with kindness, come back to the breath.

If you become aware of feelings, tension, or other intense physical sensations, just notice them, acknowledge their presence, and see if you can make space for them. Imagine with each in-breath you are creating more space inside of you for all of you, and see if you can welcome that as you return to the breath.

You may notice sensations in your body and how they change from moment to moment. Sometimes they're stronger, sometimes they stay the same, and sometimes they grow weaker—it doesn't really matter what they do. Breathe calmly into and out from the sensations of any places where you feel discomfort, imagining the breath moving into, and out from, that region of the body. As you do, remind yourself that you are getting better at feeling and being with all that is you, as it is, in this moment.

Along with physical sensations in your body, you may also notice thoughts about the sensations and thoughts about the thoughts. You may notice your mind coming up with evaluations such as "dangerous" or "getting worse," or "bored." If that happens, notice those evaluations and return to the breath and the present moment, as it is. Thoughts are thoughts, physical sensations are physical sensations, feelings are feelings, nothing more, nothing less.

If you wish, you can name thoughts and feelings as you notice them. For instance, if you notice dwelling on the past, label that "a memory" and come back to the breath. Or, if you find yourself worrying about the future, label that "worry" and again, come back to the present moment, right here, right now, being with the breath. Perhaps there is judging...notice that, and then return to the present breath, bringing a quality of kindness and compassion to your experience.

Thoughts and feelings come and go in your mind and body. The breath remains in this moment. You are the observer of your experience and not what those thoughts and feelings say, no matter how persistent or intense they may be. You are the place and space for your experience. Make that space a kind space, a gentle space, a loving space, a welcome home.

As this time of formal mindful practice comes to an end, you may wish to commit to the intention of bringing this purposeful awareness of the present moment to the rest of your day. Then, when you're ready, gradually widen your attention to take in the sounds around you...and slowly open your eyes.

This exercise can be challenging to do at first. That's okay. Remind yourself that you're learning a new skill. But don't let this initial difficulty (a judgment) deter you from practicing repeatedly over the coming weeks.

To aid your progress, we suggest tracking your experiences with the exercise by downloading the Acceptance of Thoughts and Feelings Worksheet on the book website at http://www.newharbinger.com/54476. An example of how to complete the worksheet is included. Print as many clean copies as you need.

LIFE-ENHANCEMENT EXERCISES

Centering exercises, like Acceptance of Thoughts and Feelings, help cultivate your observer mind. You've already begun this practice with earlier exercises focused on breath awareness. The beauty of these exercises is their simplicity—they can be done anytime, anywhere, even while walking. Walking is something most of us do anyway, and doing so mindfully will help you learn to move with presence.

The aim is to initiate small changes in your life. These small steps will add up over time.

For this week, make a commitment to add the following activities to your to-do list:

- Practice the Acceptance of Thoughts and Feelings exercise daily.

- Engage in mindful walking throughout your day.

- Continue with any of the previous exercises, focusing on those that provide space and shift your perspective (e.g., the I Am meditation).

- Notice any resistance you may have to these practices. Pause and examine what you might be attached to—what changes would occur if anxiety and fear no longer controlled you? Some changes may be scary, as you may feel uncertain about your identity without the WAF label.

- Above all, be patient with yourself. Your challenges didn't develop overnight. Working through this book is an act of self-care, marking the beginning of a new journey in your life.

THE TAKE-HOME MESSAGE

Everything unfolds in the present moment. Thoughts, memories, feelings, and urges all emerge here. Now is where life happens, where you've experienced both joys and challenges. It's the only place where you can take action to shape your life.

But we must learn to be present. It is, as Elizabeth Lesser (2008) describes it, like learning "piano scales, basketball drills, ballroom dance class… With increasing practice, you become more skilled at the art form itself. You do not practice to become a great scale player or drill champion. You practice to become a musician or athlete. Likewise, one does not practice meditation to become a great meditator. We meditate to wake up and live, to become skilled at the art of living" (p. 97).

Ask yourself if there's enough space within you to fully embrace all aspects of yourself, exactly as you are. If not, what barriers are preventing you from accepting yourself completely? When obstacles arise, create space for them without judgment or condemnation. Approaching WAF thoughts and feelings with mindful acceptance and compassion starves them of their power. By refraining from resistance, you cool the flames of your WAFs and open yourself to new and more fulfilling life paths. You hold the reins and have control here.

Mindful Acceptance Offers a Path out of WAFs and into Life

Reflections:

- Acceptance is vital and courageous. It helps me live a life aligned with my values.

- I can acknowledge my WAFs without getting ensnared in a struggle. This will allow me to pursue what truly matters to me.

Inquiries:

- Am I willing to approach my WAFs in a gentler way with kindness and compassion?

CHAPTER 12

Self-Compassion Is the Antidote

Though we all have the seeds of fear within us, we must learn not to water those seeds and instead nourish our positive qualities—those of compassion, understanding, and loving-kindness.

—Thich Nhat Hanh

The mind and body are very much like a garden. There, you'll find seeds of fear, anxiety, dread, stress, sadness, grief, physical discomfort, and a host of other unpleasant internal experiences. But this garden also includes the seeds of joy, peace, contentment, friendship, values and dreams, healing, kindness, love, and self-compassion.

Every human being has a garden like this, containing seeds of light and darkness. Because of that, everyone has the capacity to thrive and suffer. This capacity is not due to the presence of the seeds but with what seeds you nurture and how you tend your garden. If you nurture seeds of pain and negativity, they will grow and crowd out the positive qualities you long for in life. You must learn to water the positive qualities and not give energy to seeds of negativity and fear. How? By developing your capacity for self-kindness and self-compassion. This is one of the most powerful ways to cultivate genuine happiness.

Instead of spending time pruning the weeds of negativity in your emotional garden, you decide to give them no attention. What you put your attention on will grow greater in your awareness and thereby stronger in your life. This is what all Eastern wisdom traditions teach. So put your attention on your values, goodness, and success instead of anxiety and fear. That's how you'll grow and thrive.

When you're hurting, your natural impulse is to struggle to find comfort and relief, which only makes things worse. The harder path in these situations is to respond to your pain and woundedness with the same kindness and care you would give to others when they, like you, suffer. Self-compassion requires strength and courage to confront your vulnerabilities and face life's challenges with kindness and resilience.

As this healing response becomes more of a habit in your life, you'll find that anxiety and fear will have less power to control and limit you and your life.

THE NATURE OF SELF-COMPASSION

When you show compassion for others, what do you do? You show concern. You listen. You offer comfort and kindness. And above all, you do something good for them. You may also see part of yourself in another person who, like you, experiences pain in life and has the capacity to suffer.

In this way, compassion refers to a basic kindness for others and the wish to help ease their suffering. Notice compassion combines kindness with action. It works the same way when you show compassion for yourself.

That said, self-compassion is often misunderstood, leading to misconceptions about its nature and practice. To gain a deeper understanding of self-compassion, it's essential to clarify what it is not.

What Self-Compassion Is Not

- **Self-compassion is not self-pity:** Self-pity involves wallowing in feelings of victimization or self-indulgence, often accompanied by a sense of hopelessness or helplessness. In contrast, self-compassion involves acknowledging your pain or suffering with kindness and understanding, without getting stuck in a cycle of negativity or self-victimization. While self-pity tends to reinforce feelings of isolation and powerlessness, self-compassion fosters resilience and emotional well-being in the face of difficulty.

- **Self-compassion is not self-indulgence:** You may confuse self-compassion with self-indulgence or self-centeredness, believing that it involves prioritizing your needs and desires above others at all costs. However, self-compassion is not about prioritizing your needs at the expense of others, nor is it about indulging in selfish or hedonistic behaviors. Rather, it involves recognizing and honoring your humanity, sense of interconnectedness with other human beings, and your own well-being. This will allow you to show up for others—and yourself—with kindness, empathy, and generosity.

- **Self-compassion is not self-esteem:** While self-compassion and self-esteem share some similarities, they're distinct concepts. Self-esteem—or a subjective evaluation of your worth or value—often develops based on external validation, such as achievements or social approval, leading to fluctuations in self-worth based on external factors. In contrast, self-compassion is based on an intrinsic sense of self-worth and acceptance, independent of external validation. While self-esteem can be fragile and contingent upon success or failure, self-compassion provides a more stable and unconditional foundation for well-being.

- **Self-compassion is not resignation:** In a culture that emphasizes self-improvement and personal development, some may view self-compassion as complacency or resignation. However, self-compassion is not about settling for mediocrity or avoiding growth and change. Instead, it provides a supportive framework for your personal growth and development by fostering resilience, self-awareness, and emotional balance. Rather than striving for perfection or avoiding failure, self-compassionate people are more willing to take risks and learn from their experiences.

- **Self-compassion is not a feeling:** Many people think that self-compassion is a positive feeling, and then end up waiting for that feeling to arrive before they act in self-compassionate ways. This often keeps people stuck in their pain and suffering. You do not need to feel any particular way to give yourself self-compassion. In fact, the time to give yourself this basic kindness and care is when you're hurting or feeling lousy. So, the only feeling you need to attend to is your pain. These are your clues to act with self-compassion.

As you can see, self-compassion is distinct from self-pity, self-indulgence, self-esteem, self-improvement, weakness, and selfishness. Through practice and awareness, you can harness the healing potential of self-compassion to navigate life's challenges with greater resilience, kindness, and well-being.

What Self-Compassion Is

Self-compassion is a choice to respond to your WAFs with kindness and loving care, guided by the intention to prevent or alleviate any needless suffering. This includes whatever your mind, body, and emotions offer you. When you choose to meet any negative energy with kindness, you transmute it. This process will help you experience all forms of discomfort as an experience you share with all human beings. This will ease your suffering and help you make space for more life-affirming choices.

Self-compassion is acceptance of yourself with qualities of kindness, warmth, and understanding, especially in times of difficulty or failure. Dr. Kristin Neff—a leading self-compassion researcher—breaks self-compassion down into three main components: self-kindness, common humanity, and mindfulness. Although these components work together, they can also be used alone to cultivate a compassionate stance toward oneself, fostering resilience, emotional well-being, and personal growth.

Let's take a closer look at these fundamental features:

- Self-kindness—perhaps the most practical aspect of self-compassion—involves treating yourself with the same warmth, care, and support that you would offer to a close friend or loved one. You extend empathy for your own suffering or shortcomings rather than responding with harsh self-criticism or judgment. Practicing self-kindness involves acknowledging and validating your emotions and experiences. For example, instead of berating yourself for making a mistake, you might offer words of comfort and encouragement, recognizing that mistakes are a natural part of being human.

- Common humanity in the context of self-compassion means recognizing that suffering, flaws, and imperfections are universal aspects of the human experience. It involves understanding that everyone encounters challenges, setbacks, and difficulties at various points in their lives. You realize that you're not alone in your struggles. This perspective helps to counter feelings of isolation and inadequacy, fostering a sense of compassion toward yourself and others. Instead of viewing personal difficulties as evidence of personal failure, common humanity recognizes that failing at times is part of the broader human condition.

- Mindfulness (as you learned in chapter 11) involves maintaining a present-centered awareness of your thoughts, feelings, and bodily sensations without getting caught up in judgment. You observe the present moment with openness and curiosity, allowing experiences to arise and pass without clinging to them or pushing them away. In the context of self-compassion, mindfulness enables you to approach inner experiences with acceptance and nonreactivity rather than getting caught up in self-critical or self-doubting thoughts. By cultivating mindfulness, you'll develop greater emotional resilience in response to stress and a deeper sense of self-awareness and self-understanding.

These three components of self-compassion are interconnected and mutually reinforcing. When you practice self-kindness, you recognize your intrinsic worthiness and treat yourself with care and understanding. By acknowledging your common humanity, you cultivate a sense of connection and empathy toward yourself and others, realizing that imperfection is an integral part of the human experience. Through mindfulness, you develop the capacity to observe your inner experiences with greater clarity and equanimity, fostering emotional well-being.

EXERCISE: Traveling with Your Anxiety Child

What if anxiety looked like the child in the cartoon below—or what if it looked like your own child?

Perhaps you could treat this WAF child as you would a child of your own if they were acting out and being noisy. Think about how you might respond.

Some parents deal with the pulsating energy of their kids by lashing out, screaming at them or punishing them. The kids bear the brunt of this unfettered negative energy, and many rebel and find ways to fight and resist, in turn.

Other parents opt for a softer, yet firm, approach. They don't resort to fighting or yelling, or other punishing behavior when their child is behaving badly. They see through their own impulse to react with negative energy, and instead they redirect, refocus, and reconnect. They see their child as part of them. They wish for their child to know kindness and love, and so they respond in a way which shows that.

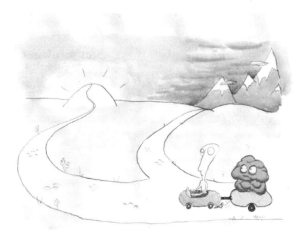

So what's your parenting strategy with your anxiety "children"? Do you yell, scream, or struggle with them? If this is what you do, has it worked, or do you end up feeling worse while your anxiety children keep acting up?

Perhaps it's time to refocus, reconnect, and redirect. After all, your WAF children are a part of you. What would it be like for you to treat your WAF children with kindness and love? You'd be firm. You wouldn't become tangled up in their wild antics or allow them to sidetrack you. You'd also take your anxiety children with you, as you do what you've set out to do.

Are you willing to do this with your anxiety children, taking them with you as you drive toward your values?

PRACTICE KINDNESS AND TENDER LOVING CARE

We've found that people with anxiety disorders are very hard on themselves. Many harbor intense self-criticism, feeling frustrated by the limitations that anxiety and fear have imposed on their lives.
Some may also get caught in the self-blame game, questioning why they can't just "get over it," and end up getting caught in cycles of anger at themselves and the world. Those with PTSD often struggle with daily anger directed toward others or themselves. They may also experience shame and regret for their actions or inactions during the traumatic event.

All this blaming and hating doesn't solve your anxiety problem. In fact, it creates the conditions for the problem to get worse. You probably know as much from your experience. What is needed here is for you to decide, perhaps for the first time, to shift your approach. Instead of blaming and hating, choose to care for your mind, body, emotional life, and anything else that your old history throws at you.

Practicing acts of kindness toward yourself and others is a great behavioral antidote to anxiety, anger, regret, shame, and even depression. This practice will make it easier for you to stop fighting with your mind and body. It's a simple thing you can do to bring more peace and joy to your life.

How to Be Kind to Yourself

Here's a powerful starting point: pledge to perform at least one act of self-kindness daily. Embrace this commitment each morning, brainstorming ways to prioritize your own care.

Acts of self-kindness are particularly important during challenging moments of fatigue, stress, or longing for comfort. In such moments, it's important to respond with TLC, or tender loving care, such as taking time to practice meditation, read a portion of a good book, go for a walk, listen to music, work in the garden, or prepare a tasty meal. You do this not because you deserve it but "just because." By nurturing yourself with tender loving care, you can overcome life's hurdles and cultivate a deeper sense of fulfillment.

Compassion is about actively choosing to care for yourself and others. It's about putting an end to self-criticism and about being your own advocate. If you're prepared to take this step, solidify your commitment by writing it down or, even better, share it with someone close to you. Let your intention to cultivate compassion wash over you and ripple out into the world.

Being kind to yourself and valued living are closely related. Whenever you do something that moves you closer to one of your values, you're also being kind to yourself. Return to your Life Compass from chapter 6 and identify something you can do, however small, in the service of one of your values. Write it down in the space below. Then commit to doing it. Make giving yourself tender loving care every day a priority.

_____

_____

Create a Compassionate Inner Landscape

In the next exercise, we'd like to guide you in transforming your inner landscape into a kind and nurturing sanctuary. The point is not to change what's already in your history but to change how you respond to that history. Listen in and access the audio version of the exercise at http://www.newharbinger.com/54476 to begin cultivating a kinder space within yourself.

EXERCISE: Loving-Kindness Meditation

Loving-kindness is soft and gentle. It is how you might handle a newborn child or the way you might touch and hold something fragile. In those moments, you open up and, with the greatest care, handle what you're given. You can do the same with anxious thoughts, worry, fears, and painful memories. There is great strength and power in kindness.

Start by getting comfortable in your kind space. Sit upright, feet flat on the floor, arms and legs uncrossed, and palms facing either up or down and resting gently on your legs. Close your eyes and bring your attention to your breath as you've done with other exercises.

Continue to focus on each gentle inhale and exhale, simply noticing the rhythm of the rising and falling of your chest and belly. As you follow the soft flow of your breath, imagine a halo of kindness sweeping over you. It starts at your head and slowly moves, ebbing and flowing, past your face and then on to your chest and belly.

As it passes, feel the energy from the halo connecting with your heart. And, as it slowly passes down your head and trunk, silently say to yourself on each inhale, *Softening, opening, allowing, welcoming, kind, peaceful, and strong*. Continue as the halo gradually sweeps down past your hips, and with each rich inhale, silently say to yourself, *I am here now—awake, alert, spacious, and alive*. As the halo sweeps over your knees, repeat with each inhale: *Softening, opening, allowing, welcoming, kind, peaceful, and strong*. When the halo reaches your toes, continue as you've done before, but this time connect with the words *I am complete, I am whole, I am*. See if you can bring the intention of kind allowing to your experience as you imagine breathing in compassionate kindness.

As you do, bring to mind someone you know who is struggling and suffering. Perhaps it's a parent, a sibling, a friend, your spouse, or a coworker. It could be a child, an older person, or someone you've heard about in the news or on TV. See if you can imagine this person in the room with you now and their suffering.

Now look into your heart and into your capacity for healing and kindness. Imagine that you could extend healing to the person you're thinking about; restore this person's mind, broken body, failings, hurts, struggles, and pain; and bring about wholeness. In your mind's eye and heart, see yourself reaching out to this person and offering kindness and healing. And then, extend your arms and offer that kindness and healing as you might a gift hidden in the cup of your hands.

In your mind's eye, see yourself wiping away this person's tears and extending love. Open your arms and wrap that person in your kind embrace—extend your heart. Allow yourself to connect your kindness with this person, who is no longer alone. You are not alone. You are united in your healing. By your generous act, you are sharing your capacity for kindness and healing. Stay with this person as long as you wish.

Continue to sit quietly with this moment in time. And when you're ready, gradually widen your attention to the sounds around you. Open your eyes with the intention to extend loving-kindness to yourself and others each moment of this day.

Kindness begets kindness. Its uplifting energy will weaken the power of your judgmental WAF mind, so you are no longer stuck. Kindness waters the seeds of compassion and acceptance in you. Many people find that their capacity for loving-kindness grows over time as they practice bringing other people to mind in the loving-kindness meditation. Try bringing to mind people you respect or like, people you don't get along with, slight acquaintances, and even total strangers, as you develop this important skill.

Embrace Your Wounds with Kindness

True self-kindness starts with acknowledging and embracing your own feelings, memories, and wounds. We all carry scars from past losses, injustices, and sometimes even trauma, and when those painful emotions and memories surface, our natural inclination is to push them aside. But instead of avoiding them, seize this moment as a chance to extend compassion and acceptance to your old hurts. This is your opportunity to heal and grow stronger.

Why should you prioritize healing your wounds? Because unaddressed pain often perpetuates itself, causing further harm to you and those around you. Untreated wounds can be unwittingly passed down to your loved ones and other people in your life, perpetuating a cycle of suffering.

Consider this. When you experience physical discomfort—like stomach pains, a cut on your knee, a toothache—you instinctively attend to it with care and compassion, right? You wouldn't exacerbate the issue by being harsh or neglectful. The same principle applies to emotional wounds—those feelings of fear, panic, worry, and shame, along with anger and self-blame.

To break free from the grip of anxiety and to live more fully, you must first prioritize self-care. This entails treating yourself with kindness and extending compassion to your anxieties. Instead of buying into negative thoughts, practice gentleness with yourself, recognizing that your emotions are a part of you and deserving of care.

You have the power to nurture yourself and tend to your anxieties and wounds with loving-kindness, without relying on others. You can decide to care for your inner wounds as tenderly as you would a beloved child in need of comfort and attention. Thich Nhat Hanh (2001) developed a beautiful exercise to practice self-directed kindness and compassion, which we've adapted here. It shows how you can take care of your anxieties and inner wounds as if they were your sick baby or child needing your loving attention.

EXERCISE: Giving Yourself Loving-Kindness

Remember when you were a little child, and you had a fever? You felt bad, and a parent or caregiver came and gave you medicine. The medicine may have helped, but it was nothing like having someone there. Remember that you didn't feel better until your parent (or other loving caregiver) came and put their hand on your burning forehead? That felt so good!

To you, this hand was precious. When they touched you, comfort, love, and compassion penetrated your body. You can experience the same right now because the healing hand of your caregiver is alive in your own hand.

Go ahead and touch your forehead or chest with your hand and see that this caring person's healing touch is still there, just like it was when you were young and sick. If you have a challenging relationship with one or more of your parents, then bring to mind anyone else who left you feeling good, loved, and cared for. The kindness of this person's hand is alive in yours. Allow the energy of their loving and tender touch to radiate through your hand and into you. Bring that quality to your experience.

As with the finger-trap exercise, this is the time to take an unusual step and be open to what may happen. Notice that you can give kindness to yourself, right now and anytime, anywhere.

Practice Giving and Receiving Kindness

The key to cultivating self-kindness and compassion lies in regular practice, and what better opportunity than when you're walking and moving about during your day? This next exercise builds on the mindful walking practice you did earlier, but with an important twist. We first learned about it from Sharon Salzberg, a well-known teacher in the art of cultivating compassion and kindness, during a retreat. As you'll see, this exercise will infuse your walking with positive energy, amplifying its impact on your well-being and the world around you.

EXERCISE: Radiate Loving-Kindness as You Walk

For this practice, you'll walk at a normal pace, inside or outside. As you walk, you'll silently repeat a meaningful phrase—one that reflects a loving-kindness intention and wish for yourself. This personal kindness mantra ought to be simple and meaningful to you.

Start your phrase with the words *May I* and limit your phrase to a few words, so that it is memorable and easy to do. For instance, you may come up with a phrase such as *May I be at peace*, *May I be kind*, *May I experience joy*, or *May I be free of suffering.*

Notice that the phrase starts with "May I," and not "I want" or "I have." The word "want" means lack and is a setup to struggle to get what you're missing. So, when you say to yourself, *I want peace*, you're affirming that you lack peace. However, you never really lack the capacity for peace or kindness; what you may lack is regular practice with peace and kindness.

Starting your phrase with "I have" can feel inauthentic and may conjure up other harsh words that are the opposite of what you're intending to do here. For instance, saying to yourself, *I have peace*, when your experience is anything but peaceful may lead your mind to protest with words like *My life is chaotic...stressed...I've never felt peace.* If you buy into these unkind reactive thoughts, you may feel worse and give up on the practice.

So, before moving on, check in with yourself. What kind and healing words resonate with you personally? Go inward and check in with your heart. Once you have the words, write them down below.

May I _____ .

May I _____ .

As you walk and move about your day, silently repeat your personal loving-kindness phrase. And when you find your attention being pulled by something or someone outside of you, gently bring your awareness to whatever it was that caught your attention, and then silently extend your personal phrase to that object, person, or creature.

For instance, if a tree caught your attention, you would then silently extend your phrase to that tree, *May this tree be at ease*. If it's a stranger, do the same. If it's a memory, thought, or feeling, do the same. If it is an animal, a car, or some other object, do the same. If this seems odd or strange, thank your mind for that thought and continue extending the phrase to anything that grabs your attention.

After you silently extend your personal loving-kindness intention to whatever grabbed your attention, bring your awareness back to yourself, and continue to walk as you repeat your personal kindness mantra silently to yourself, *May I...* Repeat this process of extending your phrase to yourself, and then to anything that pulls your attention, for as long as you wish.

This practice is a simple and powerful way to bring loving-kindness intentions into your daily life. It's best to do with an open mind and without the expectation of any immediate outcomes. Over time and with practice, loving-kindness will become more of a habit in your daily life.

So are you willing to give this a shot? If so, then set an intention to practice this exercise as often as you can while you're walking during your day. Transform your daily walks into a powerful practice of spreading loving-kindness. With each step, embody and share compassion toward yourself and others.

Later, if you like, you can extend this exercise to times when you find yourself sitting or waiting in line.

To add to your self-compassion–building toolkit, we'd like to wrap up this chapter with a self-affirmation exercise. Mirror affirmations like this one were popularized and promoted by Louise Hay, an influential author and motivational speaker in the self-help and personal development field. Grounded in principles of self-affirmation and mindfulness, this practice encourages you to cultivate self-acceptance and a compassionate inner dialogue with yourself while looking into your eyes in the mirror.

EXERCISE: Cultivate Self-Compassion Through Self-Reflection

Find a quiet and comfortable space where you can sit or stand in front of a mirror without distractions. Then, take a few deep breaths to center yourself and bring your attention to the present moment.

When you're ready, gently gaze into your own eyes in the mirror, maintaining a soft and relaxed focus. Begin by offering yourself a genuine smile, acknowledging your presence with warmth and acceptance.

Next, take a moment to reflect on a recent challenge or difficulty you've experienced, allowing yourself to feel any emotions that arise without judgment.

Now, speak to yourself with kindness and compassion, using affirming phrases that resonate with you. You can come up with your own words, or adapt the phrases below:

- "I am worthy of love and acceptance, just as I am."

- "I acknowledge my struggles with kindness and understanding."

- "I forgive myself for any mistakes or shortcomings, knowing that I'm only human."

- "I embrace myself with compassion and tenderness."

Repeat these affirmations aloud or silently, allowing them to sink in as you continue to gaze into the mirror at your eyes.

Notice any resistance or discomfort that arises, and gently remind yourself that it's okay to feel vulnerable. Offer yourself the same compassion you would offer to a dear friend in need or even a beloved pet.

As you continue to affirm yourself, observe any shifts in your inner experience. Notice if feelings of self-compassion, warmth, and acceptance begin to emerge.

Take as much time as you need with this practice, allowing yourself to fully immerse in the experience of self-compassion.

Then, when you feel ready, gradually release your gaze from the mirror and take a moment to reflect on your experience. Notice any insights or feelings that have emerged during the practice.

Finally, express gratitude to yourself for dedicating this time to nurture your inner well-being and cultivate self-compassion.

Mirror affirmations offer a powerful opportunity to cultivate self-compassion by engaging in a compassionate inner dialogue with yourself. At first this exercise may feel difficult or awkward, but if you stick with it, you'll begin to notice positive shifts within yourself. By practicing kindness, acceptance, and understanding toward yourself, you'll deepen your connection to your own inner wisdom and capacity to live in alignment with your heart and deepest longings. Through regular practice, mirror affirmations can become a valuable tool for building self-compassion and enhancing overall well-being.

LIFE-ENHANCEMENT EXERCISES

Focus on nurturing a new relationship with your anxious mind and body. Make an intention to be patient and kind with yourself, and practice acts of kindness for yourself daily, which includes making time for the important work you're doing with this workbook.

Look for ways to uphold your values as an act of kindness toward yourself and your life. Remember this is where you have control. Also work to practice letting go of resistance and struggle with your mind, emotions, and physical body. Instead, meet that negative energy with the healing power of self-compassion. This itself is also an act of self-kindness.

For this week, expand your self-care to-do list with a deeper focus on practicing exercises that nurture tender loving care toward yourself and your WAFs:

- Starting now, do something kind for yourself every day—however small that something may be.

- Be kind to your WAFs by practicing kindness and compassion toward your feelings, thoughts, memories, and hurts. You can do this by continuing to practice the Acceptance of Thoughts and Feelings exercise from chapter 11, and practice at least one loving-kindness exercise from this chapter every day. Focus on the ones that appeal most to you. As you make self-compassion a daily habit, self-kindness will come more naturally.

- Integrate acceptance and self-compassion in your daily life by continuing to label uncomfortable thoughts and feelings without getting tangled up in them. When these thoughts and feelings show up, notice them, label them, let them be, and move on with whatever you were doing. Chapter 13 will also teach you how to practice WAF surfing when emotions become intense.

THE TAKE-HOME MESSAGE

Although WAFs may feel like monsters, they're more like kids. Like children, they respond better to kindness and nurturing than to reprimands, rebukes, or harsh punishment. Practicing acceptance of your thoughts and feelings instead of trying to get rid of them is a compassionate response that will yield better results. Through daily acts of kindness toward yourself, no matter how small, you'll pave the way for self-kindness to become an ingrained habit. As self-compassion and self-kindness become second nature, they'll diminish the ability of anxiety, panic, fear, and worry to sidetrack you. This transformation will give you freedom and space to move toward your aspirations and living your values.

Responding to My Anxiety with Self-Compassion

Reflections:

- Anxiety isn't really my enemy; it's a call for self-compassion. I can empower myself by embracing kindness and understanding toward my own struggles, while recognizing that I am not alone in my pain.

- Both kindness and compassion are shown by my actions—how I engage with my thoughts, body, and existence—leading to healing and progress with or without anxiety.

Inquiries:

- Am I ready to greet my WAF children with warmth and empathy?

- Am I willing to extend kindness and self-compassion to myself, unlocking the path to reclaiming control over my life?

CHAPTER 13

Breaking Free from Anxiety

In order to be successful in life, you have to get off the couch, get out of your comfort zone, and you have to be comfortable with being uncomfortable.

—David Goggins

Resisting the natural flow of your experience holds you back and keeps you small. There may even be some comfort in remaining where you are with your anxieties and fears. After all, this is what's familiar to you. But you'll never grow that way. To grow, you need to stop resisting the flow of your inner life. You need to decide to get comfortable with being uncomfortable. This is where the magic happens!

You decide that you no longer wish to remain small, stuck in the anxiety management and control trap. Instead, you choose to grow and expand. You decide that your life is worth the investment of your time. No more fighting or struggling. No more coping with your WAFs just to get by. No more waiting for your life to begin. It's time to let go of all the needless struggle and resistance, once and for all, to make room for the life you wish to have. This much you can control. This is your moment to reclaim power and write your own narrative.

This moment of blossoming is an expression of who you are and what you care about. Every step forward is a testament to your authenticity and commitment to yourself and your values. As you reveal your true self to the world, you sow the seeds of fulfillment.

One reader, recounting his journey, shared, "The agony of avoidance and battling my anxiety surpassed the discomfort of facing it head-on and letting it be there." Embracing willingness and vulnerability, he used the tools within this workbook to navigate his path. You possess that same capacity for transformation.

Earlier chapters have revealed that you don't want your life to revolve around constant battles with WAFs. The exercises in this book have helped you uncover your core values and begin to respond to WAFs in new life-affirming ways. Now it's time to start taking first steps in the directions that truly matter to you.

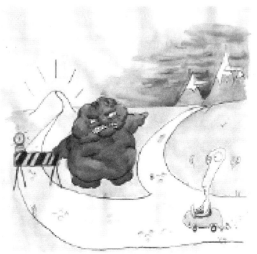

You might wonder, "What about my anxiety? Won't it block my path if I pursue my desires?" It's like facing the anxiety monster depicted in the drawing. It looks like it stands between you and your desired direction in life, causing distress. But this is an illusion.

You, not your anxiety, are the architect of your destiny. You hold the power to choose how you respond to fear, to past shadows, or to uncertain futures. You can either wage war against anxiety or make peace with it and take it along for the ride. From here on, our focus is on equipping you with additional skills to reclaim control over your life.

WHAT TO DO WHEN YOU'RE ANXIOUS OR AFRAID

As you're beginning to respond to your WAFs in a new way, one nagging question may be on your mind: What do I do when I'm getting anxious or afraid?

This is a natural question with a simple and challenging answer. Don't do what you've always done. Do something radically different! That's it. But notice that your mind might follow with, *Well, how do I do that?*

Here, it's important to be mindful that you're already doing something radically new with your WAFs. If you've gotten this far in the book, honestly and wholeheartedly practicing some of the exercises we've covered, you're moving in a new direction. You're becoming more skillful. The exercises in this chapter will simply build upon the skills you've been learning and practicing. Give yourself time with them.

For now, here are some tips for when you find yourself right in the middle of your WAFs.

Choose What You Do and Attend To

You can choose to attend to and listen to what your WAFs are telling you and do as they say. Or you can decide to watch all the activity from a compassionate observer perspective, without buying into it, and move with your hands and feet, guided by your values.

Acknowledge What's Happening Anyway

Anxiety happens. You have little say about when it shows up, how long it will last, or when it will arrive again. But you can choose what you do with it. You can choose to fight it, or you can choose to get curious about it, open up to it, meet it with self-compassion, and let it be. Like waves on the ocean, it will pass.

Do the Opposite

When your WAFs tell you to stay put sitting on your hands, get up. When you're compelled to turn away, get curious and lean in. When you're inclined to freeze, move anyway. When you feel like you're losing touch or find yourself lost in the past or future, just take a rich grounding breath and bring your awareness back to where you are right now. When you find yourself agitated, allow yourself to sit still with the energy inside. Doing the opposite of what your WAFs command is a powerful way to reclaim control of your life.

Be Kind and Gentle with Yourself

Above all, practice being gentle with yourself. This is not the time to go to war with your anxiety again. Being gentle and kind is the exact opposite of warfare. This is why it can be so powerful. Just don't use it with the intention to make the anxiety go away. If you use it as a means to an end, you'll likely find yourself right back where you started and in the middle of another war, except with a new set of weapons.

So, keep using some of the self-kindness and self-compassion exercises from chapter 12 to help you develop a new relationship with your mind, body, and experience. Practice the exercises with no agenda to feel better. There will be more of these exercises as you read along.

MOVING WITH BARRIERS

As you continue your journey out of anxiety and back into your life, you'll encounter various obstacles along the way. There may be some external obstacles—such as financial constraints, physical limitations, or other unfavorable conditions—yet the most persistent and challenging obstacles you'll encounter will likely be nagging thoughts, feelings, bodily sensations, or impulses related to your WAFs and your learning history more generally. These are the hurdles that have hindered your progress in the past, requiring a different approach to navigate effectively.

You can take these moments when WAFs show up as opportunities to respond in new ways. When you're pulled to be one of the pieces in the WAF game of chess, you shift to the board and the silent observer perspective. You remind yourself that you can provide space for your experiences.

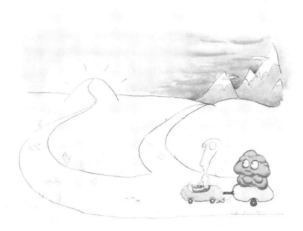

During times when you get lost in thoughts and images about the past and future, you apply mindfulness skills to return to the present moment, so you can see your experiences just as they are.

When you feel compelled to avoid or resist your WAFs in a tug-of-war, you decide to drop the rope and open up with mindful acceptance. Here, you remind yourself that your WAFs are part of you and, like all human beings, you have limited control over them. This will help you let them go and move toward living your values. Each of these WAF moments represents a pivotal point where your actions determine your path forward.

Remember that we're brought up and socialized to believe that when barriers comes up, we should get rid of or overcome them. We're also taught we can do the same with unpleasant thoughts and feelings. Hopefully, you're now beginning to see that this messaging awakens a natural inclination to struggle.

In fact, calling your anxious thoughts and feelings "barriers" or "symptoms" is probably unhelpful. Better to think of them as unpleasant experiences you share with all human beings.

So trust your lived experience over your instinct to fight against your anxious thoughts, feelings, and physical sensations. Rely on your inner wisdom rather than reactive impulses. You don't need to get rid of WAFs on your road to living your values.

The key is to accept and move *with* the barriers—take them along for the ride! You can deal with any WAF-like obstacle in the same way that you deal with other thoughts and feelings. Rather than push them aside, you make room for all the unwanted stuff that has been stopping you from doing what's best for you.

EXERCISE: Driving Your Life Bus

Imagine yourself as the driver on your Life Bus headed toward your Values Mountain, which represents _____. (Fill in the blank with one of your important values.)

As you journey forward, unwelcome and unruly passengers board your Life Bus—fear, doubt, panic, intrusive thoughts, apprehension, painful memories, and anxiety. They scream warnings and bully you, drowning out your resolve. "Don't go there! It's too dangerous. You can't handle it. You'll never be happy. Something bad will happen. STOOOPPPPP!"

You battle, trying to silence them, but eventually veer off course, feeling adrift. So you stop your bus, get out of your driver's seat, and confront them in a desperate effort to quiet them. "Shut up? Why can't you leave me alone? I'm sick of you. I just need a moment to relax."

Yet, after pouring all your attention and energy into them, you've lost sight of your destination. And nobody has left the bus!

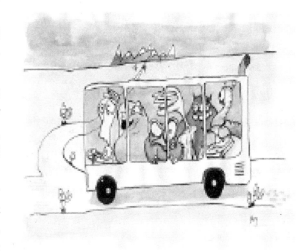

Now you're faced with a pivotal choice—you can continue wrestling with the passengers or return to the driver's seat, put your bus in gear, hold on to the steering wheel and head toward your Values Mountain.

To progress, you must remain in the driver's seat, acknowledging any passengers but without letting them dictate your journey. They'll continue to clamor for attention, but you alone must determine your course.

Be mindful that your Life Bus has other passengers that are not ominous. Amidst the chaos, you'll also find passengers reflecting your values, longing to guide you. Perhaps they've been drowned out by the other voices, but if you listen, you'll hear them. They'll remind you of the good that you're doing for your life each time you stay in the driver's seat and move your bus in directions that matter to you!

Your WAF passengers will relentlessly try to derail you—that's their job. They'll try to convince you that you don't feel like doing this anymore, that it's all too difficult, even impossible, and not worth the effort. Still, you can choose not to listen but to drive steadfastly toward your values.

Remember, you can't control the emotions or thoughts that come aboard, but you do control the direction of your Life Bus—hands on the wheel, foot on the accelerator.

Tuning In to Just So Radio

To break free from anxiety and fear, it's important to recognize that you have control over what you pay attention to and how you respond. That is, you have the power to tune in or tune out of your WAFs or your life. This choice is humorously depicted in the Anxiety News Radio metaphor by clinical psychologist Peter Thorne. When we met him, he shared an interesting comment from one of his clients. We'll call her Amy.

Before Amy came into therapy, she was most often tuned in to WANR—Anxiety News Radio—and she was sick of it. This wasn't the kind of radio most of us think of, nor was it something that Amy wanted to listen to. This radio was broadcasting from her head, and she couldn't tune it out or turn it off.

Through therapy, Amy discovered that she didn't have to remain glued to Anxiety News Radio all the time. She learned to tune in to Just So Radio with more helpful sources of information, marking the beginning of a new direction for her. Perhaps it will be for you too.

We recommend listening to the audio available at http://www.newharbinger.com/54476 with the next exercise and following along.

EXERCISE: Change the Station

Anxiety News Radio (WANR)

Here's the message you've been getting:

Welcome to Anxiety News Radio, WANR, broadcasting inside your head twenty-four hours a day, seven days a week. We're the news station you've grown up with and we're the station that never sleeps. Anxiety News Radio is known for its cutting-edge coverage of all of your deep-seated fears, worries, and all that is wrong with you. We'll offer you round-the-clock, compelling listening of doom and gloom—morning, noon, and night. Our mission is to drown out your values and keep you stuck. Our goal is to take over and control your life whenever we can. When you wake in the early hours, WANR will be there to make you aware of all the unpleasant aspects of your life, even before you get out of bed. We'll bring you all the things that you find most disturbing and distressing—anytime, anywhere. So don't forget that, and if you should try to forget us or tune us out, then we'll be sure to crank up the volume and broadcast even louder. So, please pay attention! And remember, Anxiety News Radio knows what's best for you—what you think and feel inside your skin can be really awful. So, just stay tuned and keep on listening. We know how to pull you out of your life in a flash and keep you stuck.

Just So Radio (WJSR)

Here's the message you could be tuning in to instead:

Wake Up! Anxiety News Radio is just a station—you can tune in or you can tune out! One thing is guaranteed though, whatever the time of day, you'll hear the same old stuff on WANR. If that's been really helpful to you, then go ahead, tune in and stay tuned. If not, then tune in more often to Just So Radio—WJSR. Here at WJSR, we bring you the news of actual experience, in the moment—all live, as it is, all the time. We won't bog you down with the negative spin that your mind creates, or leave you dwelling in the past or future that has yet to be. Living well right now is our business! So, at Just So Radio, we'll give it to you straight—color commentary about your experiences and your life just as they are. At WJSR, you won't find commercials trying to sell you the same old unhelpful thoughts that we know keep people stuck. Just So Radio brings you information about how things are, not how you fear they might be. At WJSR, we invite you, our listener, to step forward and touch the world, just as it is, and to touch your life, just as it is. Our business is to bring you into fuller contact with the world outside and inside your skin as we point you in directions that matter to you. And, we're entirely free! Our listeners tell us that tuning in to WJSR adds vitality to their lives and can even bring them joy. And, we get louder the more you listen to us. So stay tuned. Give us a fair trial and if you're not convinced by your own experience (please don't take our word for it), then WANR—Anxiety News Radio—is still there on the dial.

We suggest that you print the two parts of this metaphor on the front and back of a piece of paper to keep with you. That way you'll have them handy whenever you're sick of WANR and are ready to tune in to WJSR instead. Remember, what you pay attention to in your life becomes stronger and more powerful. So choose wisely!

Freeing Yourself from Mind Traps

Your mind and the simple language conventions you've learned over the years can play tricks on you that keep you stuck where you are. Recognizing them and making some simple and subtle changes in what you tell yourself can make a big difference in your life. Here's how to release yourself from two insidious mind traps: yes-butting and buying into your thoughts.

Getting Off Your But(t)s

At some point you've probably said something like "I'd like to go out, but I'm afraid of having a panic attack." Snap—you just got caught in the "yes-but" trap.

Anytime you put "but" after the first part of a statement, you undo what you just said—you negate the first part of the statement by denying it. "But" also sets up your WAFs as a barrier and problem you need to resolve before you take action. Let's see how this plays out with an example.

So when you say, "I'd like to go out, but I'm afraid of having a panic attack," you are undoing your interest in going out. The result is you'll stay home because that "but" takes the "like to go out" away.

"But" also sets you up for an internal struggle. To resolve the struggle, either the liking to go out has to go away or the fear of having a panic attack has to go away. This is why when you use buts you often end up quite literally stuck on your butt. "But" makes going out or doing much of anything impossible. If you pay close attention, you may find that you use the word "but" many times every day as a reason for not acting on your values. This unnecessarily restricts your life, holds you back, and reduces your options.

Now imagine what would happen if you replaced the word "but" with "and," as in "I'd like to go out, and I'm afraid of having a panic attack." This little change can have a dramatic impact on what might happen next. You could actually go out and be anxious and be worried all at the same time. Most importantly, you could go out and do something vital even though you might feel anxious. It would also be a more correct and honest statement of what's going on for you in the moment.

Imagine how much more space you'd have in your life if, starting today, if you were to say "and" instead of "but" every time a but is about to keep you stuck on your butt. How many more opportunities would you gain to do things? Getting off your but(t)s could be one of the most empowering things you've ever done.

Not Buying Into Your Thoughts

Buying into your thoughts feeds a good deal of suffering, and as you have learned through mindfulness practice, you can recognize thoughts and images for what they truly are. Instead of fully buying into them, you can acknowledge them as just thoughts or mental images. For instance, when you think, *I'll have a panic attack if I go out*, reframe it by telling yourself, *I'm having the thought that I'll have a panic attack if I go out*.

Or if you find yourself thinking, *If I don't learn to control my anxiety and worries, then things are going to go downhill for me*, you can even say out loud, "My mind is feeding me the message that…" This reframe more honestly and realistically describes what you're experiencing in the moment. You're having thoughts produced by your mind.

Likewise, you can apply this strategy to scary images or feelings. Label them as "picture" for images and "feelings" for emotions. For instance, you can say to yourself, *I'm having the image that I'm being attacked*. With feelings, you can say, *I'm having the feeling that _____*. Fill in the blank with whatever you typically feel.

If this feels too cumbersome, simply label thoughts as "thinking," or *Oh, there's my mind thinking*. With images, label them as "pictures," or *There's a picture*. And when physical sensations show up, label them as "sensations," or *There's a sensation of tightness in my chest*.

Practice doing this deliberately with any unhelpful thoughts your mind comes up with. This will give you space to see your thoughts for what they are: products of your mind and your history. Thoughts need not always be listened to, trusted, or believed.

Developing these new labeling and language habits may feel awkward at first. Just stay the course and keep practicing. These new skills will help you see thoughts as just thoughts, images as images, and feelings as feelings. This will give you room to move forward when your WAFs show up. Even when the most scary and intense thoughts, images, or feelings are highly believable, they're still only thoughts, images, or feelings.

It takes time to cultivate new habits. Each time you catch yourself succumbing to yes-butting or buying into your thoughts, employ these techniques. As you consistently practice, they'll create more space between you (the observer) and your mind, your experience, and your old history. This itself is change.

Riding Out Your Emotions

Imagine for a moment an ocean wave as it approaches the shore. It's steep and tall and hasn't yet crested into a breaker. Now imagine the wave nearing a group of gulls floating on the water. The birds don't fly away. They simply ride up the facing slope, round the top, and drift down the long back of the wave. That's what you can learn to do with your WAFs too.

All emotions are wavelike and time limited. They ebb and flow. Like waves, emotions build up, eventually reach a peak, and drift away. WAFs don't last forever, even if it feels like they will.

We encourage you to ride the waves of your WAFs. If you let the waves of your emotions dictate your choices, you won't get to live your life. Instead, your decisions will be at the mercy of how you feel. You know by now that there's no on-off switch for your emotions.

When Justine first came to see us, her decisions were entirely dictated by her emotions. When she felt good, she'd do something in line with her values, and when she felt bad she wouldn't do anything. You could replace emotions with upsetting thoughts too. Same deal. You'll see Justine's dilemma in the following diagram. Notice that she is entirely at the mercy of her emotional weather. You may feel that way too.

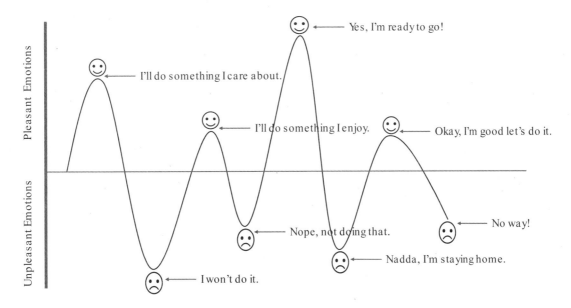

The next diagram shows why learning to ride out your emotions is so important. Notice that Justine is now willing to act, despite her emotional weather. When she feels good, she acts on her values, and when she feels uncomfortable, she still acts on her values. When you do that, you—rather than your emotions—are in charge.

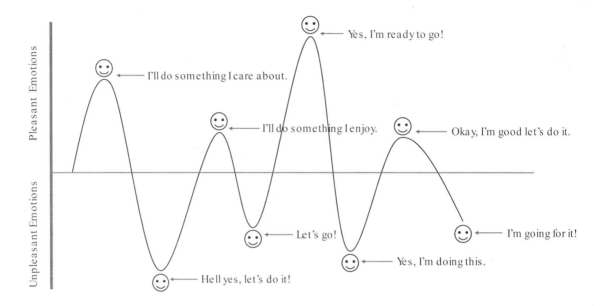

To develop this skill of willingly riding out your emotions, listen to the audio of the following exercise with your eyes closed and try to imagine the entire scene at a beach.

EXERCISE: WAF Surfing

Right now you have a chance to learn to ride the wave of your worries, anxieties, and fears—your WAFs. If you're willing, then think of a recent situation where you felt afraid, panicky, nervous, worried, or upset. Visualize the scene and remember how you felt. Pause for a while before going on.

Notice the worrying and disturbing thoughts. Perhaps you'll notice images of disaster too. Keep focusing on the upsetting scene as well as on the judgments you made about it and what was happening inside you. Let your anxiety rise to at least a 4 or 5 on a scale of 10.

Then step into the role of the observer, the part of you that can notice thoughts as thoughts, feelings as feelings, and sensations as sensations without judgment. Notice the sensations and how your mind evaluates them. Simply label them all—*I am noticing* sensations of warmth... there's another one of tightness... There's the thought that it's dangerous, that I'm losing control. Just let your body and mind do its thing. Here, you are the witness to all this activity.

Do the same with worries, other thoughts, and images that show up—the old story line. None of them are right or wrong, true or false. Label them as they arise, acknowledging their presence without trying to control or change them. Don't try to push them away either.

In your mind, you can now ride the waves of your WAFs. You must initially face their steep leading edge. At this point, the waves are tall and scary. You may feel that they'll go on forever and overpower you, or that you may drown—but remember to keep riding the feelings.

Become aware of the point where your WAF wave plateaus and begins to diminish. Embrace the slow descent, accepting where you are on the wave without rushing. It moves at its own speed—all you can and need to do is watch thoughts and sensations come and go, observing the wave's progress until it passes completely. Simply let go and allow it to carry you through.

You can watch your thoughts and bodily sensations using this observer part of yourself. You are not caught up in the wave but can just notice and experience it. Wave or not, you still have choices in how you respond. Notice also that you can notice the progress of the wave. There's nothing more to do. Keep watching until each WAF wave passes.

Using the Energy of Anxiety Wisely

Pema Chödrön (2001) describes an intriguing way you can use the energy of anxiety wisely. Emotions proliferate through our internal dialogue—what your mind is telling you about your anxiety. If you label those thoughts as "thinking" when you notice them and just observe what's going on, you may be able to sense the vital, pulsating energy beneath them. This energy underlies all of your emotional experiences, and there's nothing wrong or harmful about it.

The challenge is to stay with this underlying energy: to experience it, to leave it as it is, and, when possible, to put it to good use. When anxiety arises uninvited, let go of your old story line about it and connect directly with the energy just below the surface. What remains is a *felt* experience, not the story line your mind is feeding you about what's happening.

If you feel, and can stay with, the energy in your body—neither acting on it nor suppressing it—you can harness it in the service of actions that move you forward toward achieving your valued goals. The raw energy of anxiety is fuel. You get to choose to use that fuel for you or against you.

LEARNING TO ALLOW YOUR ANXIETY

Mindfulness exercises are a way of learning that you cannot choose what comes into your mind and what you feel. You can only choose what you pay attention to, *how* you pay attention, and what you *do*. This is how you change your relationship with your mind, body, and world.

In this next exercise, we're expanding on your existing skills by inviting you to embrace bodily sensations, unwelcome thoughts, worries, and images with acceptance and compassion. You'll work on leaning into them, like you did previously with the finger trap exercise in chapter 11.

By leaning in, you're creating room for unwanted thoughts, feelings, and sensations to exist without resistance because they're there whether you acknowledge them or not. This will create space to experience your emotions and thoughts as they truly are, not as your mind tells you they are. This space, in turn, will give you the freedom to reclaim the life you've put on hold for too long. Are you ready to take this step?

If you're willing, find a quiet place where distractions are minimal—think of this as a kind space, or haven of peace and transformation. Take your time with each section of the exercise, pausing to reflect. It will only take about fifteen minutes of your time. The easiest way to do this exercise is by listening to the audio recording. After practicing for a week or two, you may prefer to practice at your own pace without the audio.

EXERCISE: Kindly Allowing Anxiety

Go ahead and get in a comfortable position in your chair. Sit upright with your feet flat on the floor, your arms and legs uncrossed, and your hands resting in your lap (palms up or down). Allow your eyes to close gently.

Take a few moments to get in touch with your breath and the gentle rising and falling of your chest and belly. There's no need to control your breathing in any way—simply let the breath breathe itself. As best you can, also bring an attitude of kind allowing and gentleness to the rest of your experience. There's nothing to be fixed. There's nothing else to do. Simply allow your experience to be your experience, just as it is.

As you sink more deeply into this moment of just being where you are, see if you can be present with your values and commitments. Ask yourself, *Why am I here? Where do I want to go? What do I want to be about in my life?* Connect with the truth of it in your heart, and bring your awareness more fully to something you care about. Look to one of your values that has been difficult for you to act on because of barriers. Rest in the truth of your experience with each natural breath and become aware of what shows up that has been hard for you.

It could be a troubling thought, a worry, an image, or an intense bodily sensation. Gently, directly, and firmly shift your attention on and into the discomfort, no matter how bad it seems. Notice any strong feelings that may arise in your body. Allow those feelings to be as they are, and observe what your mind tells you about them. Simply hold your thoughts and feelings in awareness with a sense of curiosity and kindness. Stay with your discomfort, breathe with it, and see if you can gently open up to it and make space for it. With each new breath, imagine that you are creating more and more space for this barrier to simply be there. Simply allowing it to be as it is. Notice also who it is that is noticing all these thoughts and feelings... Can you sense your silent observer?

If you ever notice yourself tensing up and resisting, pushing away from the experience, just acknowledge that and see if you can make some space for whatever you're experiencing, with each new breath. Is this feeling or thought really your enemy? Or can you have it, notice it, own it, and let it be? Can you make room for the discomfort, for the tension, for the anxiety? What does it really feel like to allow it to be there, moment to moment? Is this something you *must* struggle with, or can you invite the discomfort in, saying to yourself, *I welcome you in because you are just a part of my experience right now?*

If the sensations or discomfort grow stronger, acknowledge that, stay with them, breathe with them, and allow them to just be. Is this discomfort something you *must not* have, you *cannot* have? Can you create space for the discomfort in your heart? Is there room inside you to feel that, with compassion and kindness toward yourself and your experience? Breathe and create more space in your heart center for you to hold all of you.

As you embrace your experience, you may notice thoughts coming along with the physical sensations, and you may see thoughts about your thoughts. You may also notice your mind coming up with judgmental labels such as "dangerous" or "getting worse." When that happens, the practice is the same. Stay with them, breathe into them, creating more and more space within you to have what you are experiencing, just as it is. Simply notice thoughts as thoughts, physical sensations as physical sensations, feelings as feelings—nothing more, nothing less.

Stay with your discomfort for as long as it pulls on your attention. If and when you sense that the anxiety and other discomfort are no longer pulling for your attention, let them go.

As this time for practice comes to a close, take a few rich inhales and slow cleansing exhales. Then, gradually widen your attention to take in the sounds around you. Take a moment to make the intention to bring this sense of gentle allowing and self-acceptance into the present moment and the rest of your day. Then, slowly open your eyes.

This exercise can be tough, especially as you're intentionally facing your WAF experiences for the first time. But don't let the challenge deter you—it gets easier with practice.

Expect a variety of outcomes too—relaxation, tension, sadness—each valid and part of the process. The goal is to become more comfortable with your anxiety-related thoughts and feelings, embracing them rather than resisting. Put another way, you're learning to honor your experience by staying with yourself just as you are.

So, go easy on yourself as you practice. Remember, the point of learning to allow and accept your anxieties and fears is to give you the freedom to move forward in your life. Acceptance empowers you to do what you really want to do along *with* whatever arises in the process.

Track your progress over the next several weeks using the Kindly Allowing Anxiety Worksheet that you'll find at http://www.newharbinger.com/54476. This worksheet will give your practice some structure; you'll also see that we've included an example of how to complete the worksheet.

LIFE-ENHANCEMENT EXERCISES

This week, dedicate time to practice the exercises outlined in this chapter, integrating them into your self-care routine. Make a point to do the Kindly Allowing Anxiety exercise at least once daily. Feel free to revisit exercises from previous chapters as well—repetition breeds mastery; what once seemed extraordinary will become ordinary with practice. So, experiment with the exercises, hone your skills, and seize every opportunity to apply them in real-life situations. Above all, stay connected to your purpose. This journey is about aligning with what truly matters to you and crafting the life you desire, even if anxiety occasionally tags along.

THE TAKE-HOME MESSAGE

Anxiety can either dominate your life or be a passing experience that comes and goes on its own, depending on how you respond to it. Your thoughts and feelings don't have to dictate your actions. You always have choices. We hope you're beginning to realize this for yourself.

Each aspect of this chapter builds upon the skills you've been cultivating throughout the book. Every moment of discomfort offers an opportunity to adopt a new approach. Keep nurturing your ability to respond with kindness, mindful observation, patience, and integrity, all while staying true to your values.

Facing and Allowing Anxiety to Reclaim My Life

Reflections:

- Emotions come and go like waves, but I can decide how I respond to them and what I am willing to do with them.

- Pain is inevitable. Avoiding WAF pain means avoiding life itself. Embracing and softening to my anxious mind and body is the key to reclaiming my life. When I do that, anxiety is no longer a barrier, but an experience I share with the rest of humanity.

Inquiries:

- Am I willing to make peace with my WAFs and kindly allow them to be just as they are and take them along on my life journey?

- Am I ready to embrace anxious discomfort when it arises, to regain control of my life?

CHAPTER 14

Disarming the Anxious Mind

If you change the way you look at things, the things you look at change.

—Wayne Dyer

Your mind can be your greatest friend and your worst enemy. It all depends on what you do with it. This chapter focuses on the transformative power of perspective and the idea that we can change how we view and respond to our lived experience. Seen in this way, thoughts are just thoughts, ethereal, without form or substance. Things that you might imagine or visualize in your mind are like that too. They can seem quite real, but when you look at them, you'll find that there really isn't much to them at all.

YOUR MIND MACHINE

Your mind is a relentless creator, churning out thoughts ceaselessly. This is the nature of being human—we all experience it. Your mind constructs, evaluates, problem-solves, and interprets your experiences. It can paint imaginary futures or drag you back into the past. It's both the instrument of love and kindness and the source of anxiety, hatred, blame, and self-loathing. Remarkable, isn't it?

Your mind will continue churning out thoughts as long as you're alive. There's no healthy way to unplug it or remove what's already in there. But you do have the power to choose how you engage with it. You don't have to accept everything your mind machine produces; you can observe what it does from a distance. You don't have to take the bait.

Below, you'll find an exercise from our colleague Richard Whitney, which will give you a better sense of what we mean.

EXERCISE: Unhooking Your Judgmental Mind

Our minds work like a fly fisher whose job it is to catch trout by tricking them into taking the bait. Good fly fishers take time to match their artificial flies to the insects that trout are feeding on. And they carefully present those flies with each cast.

When they get it right, the trout can't tell the difference between a real insect and the fake fly. The trout sees it floating by, buys that the fly is real, bites, and gets hooked. The trout then finds itself in a fight for its life.

Now imagine that you are a trout, and your mind is a skilled fly fisher, creating thoughts, worries, and images that look like carefully crafted flies—the ones you'll bite on. Your mind casts them out onto the stream of life, again and again, here, there, and just about anywhere.

They seem so real that you bite and get hooked. Perhaps you get hooked on the wingless phobic or the blue-winged panicker or the soft-hackled worrier. You may even get snared by the hopeless dun, the out-of-control dragonfly, or the mad-and-angry streamer. Once you're hooked, there's nothing left to do but struggle. The struggle sets the hook deeper. You're now in a fight for your life, being pulled in directions you don't want to go.

There's one important difference between a fly fisher and your mind, however. Your mind has barbless hooks. Your mind will tell you there is a barb on the hook and that you can't get off, and it may feel like you can't get off. But if you stop struggling and observe the hook more closely, you'll see that the hook has no barbs. You can let go and set yourself free.

In the river of life, WAF flies constantly drift by, tempting you with their barbless hooks. With practice, you'll become adept at recognizing them for what they are: *Oh, that's just another WAF fly floating by; I don't have to bite.* This will reduce the likelihood of your getting hooked by unhelpful thoughts.

Occasionally, your mind will deceive you, and you'll find yourself biting. It's a natural part of the human experience. The key lies in noticing when you've been hooked. Once you recognize it, you have the power to choose to let go and swim on.

Thoughts Are Just Words Too

Our minds tend to take words literally, and before we know it, the thought has become the real thing in our mind—no longer just a thought or words. If we can step back a little and begin to notice the thought as just a bunch of words, we can open our minds to more than the automatic conclusion we draw from those words.

This next exercise, inspired by an activity developed by our colleagues Matthew McKay and Catherine Sutker (2007), will help you see for yourself that thoughts are just words.

EXERCISE: Demoting Your WAF Mind Playfully

Let's start with the word "spider." What image does it conjure in your mind? Can you visualize it crawling? If spiders evoke fear or disgust for you, acknowledge those sensations. Now, position yourself near a clock. Repeat the word "spider" aloud rapidly for exactly forty seconds.

When you're done, consider how the word "spider" changed in meaning after forty seconds. Did it still evoke feelings of creepiness, if it did initially? Did the image of the spider persist? Did the words begin to blur together? For many, the word transforms into a mere sound—"ider, ider, ider..."—and its meaning fades during those forty seconds.

This exercise illustrates how the judgmental mind can create WAF monsters that are illusions. These monsters are simply words linked with images and sounds, carrying meanings we assign to them. Understanding this aspect of language will allow you to change your relationship with unpleasant thoughts, feelings, and images. You might even begin to take your thoughts less seriously.

Right now, go back to your Valued Directions Worksheet and Life Compass from chapter 6. Look at one of your important values and the WAF barriers that seem to stand in the way. Select a barrier and give it a one-word name, like "worry," "panic," "anxiousness," "aloneness," "uncertainty," "airplane," "sadness," "death," "dirtiness," "sickness," "heights," "crashes," or "trapped." Feel free to pick a negative word that you think about yourself, like "unattractive," "stupid," "worthless," or "boring." It might even hurt or make you mad to think this word.

Now repeat that word out loud as fast as you can for about forty seconds. After that, does it still sound as believable? Can you see how it's also just a word, a sound with no meaning or truth?

You can create even more space by doing the following: say the thought out loud and slowly, like "wooooooorrrrrryyyy," "stuuuuupid," or "unreeeeeal." Say it in another voice—as a child or an old person, as Minnie Mouse or Donald Duck, as someone intoxicated, or as a grumpy person. Notice what happens as you add a playful quality to the thoughts.

To add another layer of play, you can put your thought to music. Take the thought and sing it to yourself. Put it to the melody of a favorite holiday tune, children's song, or whatever song you'd like. Start with something simple like "Jingle Bells" or "Row, Row, Row Your Boat." See what happens to the thought as you put it to music.

These exercises can be done anytime or anywhere. As you practice them, you'll strengthen your ability to disengage from negative hooks and to view thoughts, evaluations, and self-narratives as mere mental constructs. Some of them might even make you laugh.

Your Mind as a Person

We've all met people we didn't like. You have too. They may annoy you. They may even scare you, revealing your deepest fears and vulnerabilities. Their words and actions are unwelcome and hurtful, leaving you feeling bad.

Your mind can be like one of these people—bullying and taunting you with its unwelcome labels, criticisms, and predictions. Here, you can benefit from getting some perspective. Simply asking yourself, *Who's telling me that right now?* is a good starting point. You might answer, *I'm telling me that, but are you really?* Are you reducible to your mind's epithets, or is there more to you than what you think? Recall, there's a part of you that can observe, and there's part of you that identifies with your learning history. You can choose to be the witnessing observer rather than identify with your mind.

We understand that looking at thoughts instead of from them is hard for many people. The next exercise, created by John's wife, Jamie, emerged naturally during her therapeutic work with individuals struggling with anxiety and depression. We share it with you because it can help create space between you and your mind's unhelpful negative narratives.

> *Your mind is not always your best friend.*

EXERCISE: Personifying Your WAF Mind

Begin by tuning in to the unsettling messages your WAF mind feeds you about you and your life before, during, or after you're anxious or afraid. Now, imagine this WAF mind were a person you just met. Or, alternatively, think of your mind as a made-up character or creature. The only rule here is that your mind cannot be you—it's only a part of you.

On a separate piece of paper, describe what this person is like. Start with your mind's personality. What kind of personality does your WAF mind have? What kind of person are you dealing with here? Is this a caring, loving person? Is this someone you'd like to spend time with? Would you want to be friends or have this person over for dinner?

Once you have the personality of your WAF mind down, fill in some details. Do they have a gender, and if so, what is it? How old are they? Describe this person's appearance. For instance, how tall are they? What does their face and body look like? What do they wear? Are they well-groomed or unkempt? How does this person carry themselves?

Now go further. How does this person sound? Loud? Opinionated? Boastful? Negative? Nagging? Does the person speak with an accent?

Get it all down in a paragraph or two. And once you have it, stop and read what you wrote down. Who is this mind of yours? Give it a name, even a funny one, and then pause to reflect.

When you look at the WAF character you just created, do you really want to hang out with them? Do you need to listen to everything they say or command you do?

When Lisa, a bank teller, did this exercise, she identified several tormenting WAF messages: "You're worthless," "You can't do anything right," "You're broken—damaged goods," "You can't do it," "You're unlovable," "You'll freak out," and "You're too anxious to do anything." She then created a character who embodied her WAF mind and created a made-up name for it—Sir Widgerton. After personifying her WAF mind, Lisa quickly realized she didn't want to spend her time listening to Sir Widgerton's negative chatter or following its orders. In fact, she felt sorry for her mind, recognizing it as a sad, bitter, and miserable character who lived in a chronic state of fear and negativity.

Lisa experienced a profound shift of perspective. She saw her WAF mind as an unhelpful character that she didn't have to spend time with or listen to. From then on, whenever Lisa experienced unhelpful WAF thoughts, she told herself, "There's Sir Widgerton again, off on another doom and gloom rant trying to bring me down."

Over time, she began to catch Sir Widgerton showing up uninvited instead of seeing her thoughts as something she must always believe or identify with. This shift in perspective, along with a newfound lightness, humor, and compassion for Sir Widgerton, offered Lisa a newfound sense of freedom.

Embracing Uncertainty

Intolerance of uncertainty is a common concern and one that often accompanies anxiety and fear. We humans don't like being in a place of not knowing, particularly about bad things that could happen in the future. This is where the mind jumps in.

Right now, you can think about what you'll be doing tomorrow around dinnertime. You can also think about what will happen five days from now. If we push, you might even be able to tell us what your life may be like ten or twenty years from now.

Here, it's important to notice that you're having thoughts about the future. You do not know the future. Nobody has that kind of crystal ball. But your mind can fool you into thinking that you do, and if your thoughts involve anxiety, that future looks bad. Your mind says, *When you go to the grocery store this afternoon, you're going to freak out and make a fool of yourself!*

Or, if you've been invited to a social gathering this coming weekend, your mind might claim, *Everyone will be judging you because you're so awkward…and you're going to say something stupid and embarrass yourself.*

If you struggle with obsessions, your mind will tell you things like *If you don't say the numbers and do the routine, bad things are going to happen to your kids.* Again, these are thoughts about an unknown future.

When your anxious mind feeds you foreboding thoughts and images about the unknowable future and you buy into them, you'll have something to be anxious about. This is the problem with worry. Remember, worry is about the future.

So, when you think, *I'm going to have a panic attack on the way to work tomorrow*, you have just told yourself that you will have a panic attack. Your worrying mind has just resolved any uncertainty by claiming that it knows you will have one.

A more honest response here is that you're having thoughts about the future, and you can never know exactly what the future holds. You may have a panic attack, or you may not. Bad things could happen to your kids, or they may not. That's the truth. You just don't know.

The more you embrace this basic truth about life and the human experience, the less you'll find yourself worrying about what may or will happen. This will help you focus on what you can do now to live your life.

We recommend listening to the audio at http://www.newharbinger.com/54476 with the next exercise and following along.

EXERCISE: Practice Embracing Uncertainty

Find a comfortable space where you can sit or lie down without distractions. Once you're settled, take a few deep breaths to center yourself. Then reflect on a future situation or decision that leaves you feeling worried and anxious.

Notice any physical sensations, emotions, or thoughts that may arise as you think about this situation. Allow yourself to sit with these feelings and thoughts without judgment or resistance. As you do, imagine yourself surrounded by a warm comforting light, radiating from within you.

With each natural breath, imagine letting go of the need for certainty and control. Notice how your mind tells you that things will go terribly, horribly wrong. Acknowledge these thoughts are about the future; they're not the future itself. Embrace the truth that uncertainty is a natural part of life, and it can lead to growth and discovery. Then, let any future thoughts and dire predictions go with each exhale.

When you begin to shed catastrophic and dark thoughts about the future, you may shift into repeating a calming affirmation silently to yourself, such as *I trust in the process of life. I am capable of handling whatever comes my way.* Or, *I have no idea how things will go or turn out, and I am willing to be present and do what I can now to make a difference in my life.*

Continue as long as you wish. Then, when you're ready, slowly open your eyes and return to the present moment. Set the intention to bring this sense of peace and acceptance of uncertainty into your daily life.

Your Mind Machine and Your Values

At times, your mind is your greatest ally, but at other times it can be your worst enemy. To distinguish between the two, begin by noticing what your mind is telling you, then ask yourself three simple questions based on your lived experiences, not the false promises your mind creates:

If I listen to and do what my inner voice tells me right now:

1. Will I do more or less with my life in this moment?

2. Does it leave me feeling better or worse?

3. Will it move me toward or away from my values?

If you answered less, worse, and away, and you still do what your mind says, then you won't move forward. You'll remain hooked, struggling, and stuck.

So, what's the solution? It's to take a radically different approach. Practice mindful compassion by observing your mind's hooks and choosing not to get entangled in them. The next exercises will help you do more of that.

FEEL EXERCISES TO UNHOOK YOUR JUDGMENTAL MIND

FEEL—Feeling Experiences Enriches Living—exercises build on everything you've been learning up to this point. The thought and imagery exercises that comprise the rest of this chapter offer opportunities to detach from your anxious judgmental mind and respond with kindness. We encourage you to explore all the exercises to learn a new skill set. It's fine if just a few truly resonate with you, but you'll need to allow yourself time with each exercise before deciding which ones suit you best.

You can use the following worksheet to track your progress with the FEEL thought and imagery exercises in this chapter. As you do, take time to review your responses to each exercise over time and look for changes in a positive direction, especially with willingness, struggle, and avoidance. For further structure, you may want to refer to "How to Do FEEL Exercises in Eight Simple Steps" in chapter 15 (in steps 5 and 8, use the FEEL Thought and Imagery Worksheet). Both the worksheet and these eight simple steps are available at http://www.newharbinger.com/54476.

FEEL* Thought and Imagery Worksheet

Instructions: Write down the date and time after completing the exercise, and record your reactions under each category.

Date: _____ Time: _____ a.m./p.m.

0	1	2	3	4	5	6	7	8	9	10
Low					Moderate					Extreme

Exercise	Sensation Intensity (Rate 0–10)	Anxiety Level (Rate 0–10)	Willingness to Experience (Yes or No?)	Struggle with Experience (Rate 0–10)	Avoidance of Experience (Rate 0–10)
Bubble Wand	_____	_____	_____	_____	_____
Kind Allowing with Disturbing Images	_____	_____	_____	_____	_____
Difficult Thoughts and Urges Cards	_____	_____	_____	_____	_____
Putting Thoughts and Urges on Cards	_____	_____	_____	_____	_____
Stand Silently with Urges	_____	_____	_____	_____	_____
Leaves on a Stream	_____	_____	_____	_____	_____
Other: _____	_____	_____	_____	_____	_____

* Feeling Experience Enriches Living

FEEL Exercise for Nagging Worries and Doubts

This imagery exercise is lengthy, and it's one of the most important exercises in this book. Set aside ten to fifteen minutes for it. We strongly suggest beginning by listening to the audio recording provided to guide your imagination. As you follow along, feel free to pause as needed. You can also read through the script a few times first, and then close your eyes to do the exercise.

EXERCISE: Bubble Wand

Get in a comfortable position in a chair. Sit upright with your feet flat on the floor, your arms and legs uncrossed, and your hands resting in your lap (palms up or down, whichever is more comfortable). Close your eyes and take a few deep breaths. Allow your body to rest without drifting off to sleep. Bring an intention of kindness to this practice.

Now, bring into your awareness a recent situation where you found yourself in a bout of endless worry. Perhaps it's a situation you know all too well or one you wrote down on your LIFE Worksheets over the past weeks.

Really work to bring this experience into your full awareness and right into the room with you. Make it as real as possible. Continue to visualize the situation until you can notice a wave of unpleasant changes sweeping over your body and mind. Allow yourself to connect with the experience. Relive every bit of it as best as you can. Keep doing so until you're at a point where you feel taken over by anxiety and tension and have a strong desire to do something about it.

Now, we want you to go more deeply into this experience. Imagine that you have a large bubble wand like the kind that kids sometimes play with at the beach or in the park. Fill the wand with bubble soap. Then look within yourself and notice all the elements of the unsettling experience. Start by locating one of the most obvious judgments or worrisome thoughts.

Take your bubble wand and sweep it through each worry thought, one by one. Trap each thought in a giant bubble. Then, notice each thought in its bubble and label it as you watch each drift upward in the gentle breeze—*There goes worrying...what if-ing...second-guessing... judging...blaming...shaming...criticizing.* Keep watching the bubbles go higher and higher until they're out of sight. Then take a few slow, deep breaths.

Allow yourself to go more deeply into this experience. See if you can find the next thought underneath the first worry. For example, if you worry about not having enough money to make ends meet, then you might gently ask, *And if that were true, then what?* Watch what your mind comes up with. Perhaps it's the thought *I won't be able to pay my bills.* Notice that thought and place it in a giant bubble and watch it float upward. Follow this with *And then what?* Keep going with an attitude of gentle curiosity and kind allowing.

As you go more deeply into your worry, you'll likely notice more physical sensations in your body: heart pounding in the chest, feeling shaky, trembling hands, shortness of breath, feeling hot, or an upset stomach. There's tension everywhere. You may feel like you're about to pop. As that unfolds, notice your impulses to respond and label these sensations one at a time: *There is my impulse to shout...run away...shut down...struggle...make a fist...lash out...point my finger...;* or stop this exercise.

Your task now is both simple and difficult: Do nothing! Sit with these thoughts, sensations, and impulses. Feel the restless energy in this situation. Sitting still and doing nothing is the last thing you want to do, and it's the wisest thing you can do. Say nothing. Do nothing. You want resolution now, and there isn't any.

The energy of anxiety and worry works like a big ocean wave—just allow yourself to ride with each wave as it comes and goes into and out of your awareness. Watch as the wave rises until it reaches its peak, staying strong and powerful for a while, and then eventually settles back down and drifts away. Continue to sit still with the energy in this situation and let the worry wave run its course.

Then gently return to the worry situation and take a final inventory. What are you left with here? What do you see? If you look closely, you'll see two things: the pain and hurt that fueled your worry to begin with, and your values.

See if you can turn your attention to the pain and hurt underneath the worry. Give that pain and hurt a label. If you have a hard time identifying the hurt, ask yourself, *What would I have left to feel if I didn't get caught up in worry in this situation?* Take a moment to really take stock.

Perhaps you see hurt, fear, abandonment, loneliness, inadequacy, loss, guilt, vulnerability, or shame. There is no need to trap these feelings or cover them. They're part of you and belong to you without being you or defining who you are. Just allow them to be. Make space for them.

As if they were open wounds, take care of these feelings by bringing kindness, care, and compassion to your experience and to this moment. Forgive yourself for burying and rejecting your pain for so long, for acting in ways to push it from view.

If at any time you feel like stopping and stepping back inside your worry armor, thank your mind for that option and simply return to your experience. If you notice judgment or resentment popping up again, place these thoughts into their own bubbles and let them go, floating upward.

Next, gently turn your attention to your values lying close by. Which ones do you see? Pick one or two that are important to you. Now ask yourself this question: *If worry and doubt are between me and moving in the direction of those values, am I willing to have them and still do what matters to me?* If you're willing, worry is no longer a barrier. It's just a thought.

Now think of a situation where worry got in the way of you acting in accord with your values. Then go ahead and imagine yourself doing what you value and bringing your hurt and pain with you.

That probably feels strange, and it also feels vital because you're moving toward what you care about in life. Here, you're exerting control where you truly have it. Take time to really connect with this. This is what it's all about!

Then, when you're ready, gradually widen your attention to take in the sounds around you in the room you're in. Take a moment to make the intention to bring this sense of compassion and forgiveness into the present moment and to the rest of your experience on this day.

This exercise can be challenging. At first, you may have trouble taking an observer's perspective. Don't beat yourself up over this or any "failures" or difficulties. Being compassionate isn't about perfection. Keep practicing, be patient, and be gentle with yourself. Commit to doing the exercise again tomorrow and the day after. Simply do your best.

Repeat the same worry episode once daily until you can readily adopt a silent observer self-perspective while staying with any unpleasant energy that may arise. Then, select a different worry episode and repeat the process.

Continue practicing until you can remain with bodily discomfort and hurt, with compassion and forgiveness, and with minimal entanglement in judgment. This may require several days or weeks of practice. The important thing is to stay committed to the process.

FEEL Exercise for Disturbing Images

Being able to imagine—to visualize—is a great gift. We can paint in our mind's eye portraits of experiences that once were or have yet to be, and we can do this anytime and anywhere. We can also create imaginary realities and treat them as if they were real.

Our minds can turn any word into an image, and we can also put most images into words. Think the word "sunset" and you may find yourself being able to see one in your mind. Read the word "jerk," and you may be able to visualize a person who treated you or others poorly.

You have these capacities and need them. These processes are at work both when you experience joyful and serene images and thoughts and when you experience disturbing or fearful thoughts. Here's a powerful way to learn to hold your WAF images more lightly.

EXERCISE: Kind Allowing with Disturbing Images

Start by generating a few sentences describing troublesome or disturbing WAF images. You can write in your journal or on a piece of paper. Here are a few examples:

- I'm in a car accident, hurt someone, and it was my fault.

- I'm meeting new people, and everyone is judging me.

- I'm homeless and couldn't do my job, because I'm anxious.

- I'm in a psychiatric hospital because I'm crazy.

- I'm trapped in a seat in the middle section of a crowded theater with no clear exit.

- I'm not safe and will be attacked.

- I'm not going to make it if my husband's health gets worse.

Struggling to conjure images? If so, you're not alone. If you suffered trauma, it can be challenging to remember and visualize painful events from your past. Stuck in a worry loop? If so, your mind may struggle to break free from difficult thoughts long enough for you to do this exercise. If your challenge is disturbing obsessions, then your imagery will often be dark and unwelcome. You may even fear that thoughts will come true if you think them.

We also hear some people say, "I can't do these kinds of visualization exercises." If that sounds like you, be careful. You can visualize if you have the capacity to feel anxious or afraid. If you get distressed thinking about your past, or you worry about the future, you too can visualize. If you experience obsessions and respond with fear, you also have this ability. You may not be aware that your mind is creating images and narratives, but it is and that's the fuel for anxiety and fear. You also may be applying too strict a definition of imagining. We're not asking you to come up with a picture or a movie but rather to watch what your mind tells you about events that make you anxious or afraid. If you can put this into words, you can set the scene and imagine it happening.

Whatever the reasons your mind offers about your imagined difficulties, you need to ask yourself if your reaction is serving you well or not. If you've tended to blot out or shut down thinking about upsetting images, ask yourself if not thinking about this is working for you. What does your experience tell you? Will more of the same—shutting down, closing up, or saying "I can't do it"—get in the way of your effort to change in more vital ways? Can you flip your willingness switch on? Are you willing to create that list now? If so, do it and then continue.

Once you have your list, go over it with both eyes fixed on willingness. For each image, ask whether you are 100 percent willing to have the WAF image just as it is. Remember, it's okay if you don't like it or if the image makes you uncomfortable. The willingness question is not about liking anything. The question is, are you open to having that image and the discomfort that goes along with it, without doing anything about it?

Next, get settled in a quiet space. Close your eyes and become centered on the breath. Then, when you're ready, select an image that you're 100 percent willing to have, and hold that image gently in your awareness.

Recognize the image and label it as such: *I am having the image of...* Bring kindness and compassion to the image as if you were holding something that you really care about. As you do, notice that the passengers on your Life Bus are just thoughts and images. You, not they, control the gas pedal, brake, and steering wheel. You, not they, control what you do.

Allow yourself to bring an attitude of kind allowing to the image for at least five minutes beyond the point at which the image is vivid. Then you may move on to the next image, or you can plan for your next practice. It's best to stay with one image until you can do it with your willingness switch in the on position most of the time. Then you're ready to move on to a different image.

Go through all the images you rated as ones you'd be willing to have, and then practice with the ones that you were unwilling to have. Be patient and take your time.

If you continue to have difficultly bringing kindness to your own unpleasant thoughts and images, you may use prompts from newspaper stories or look to photographs or movies to help you practice simply being with unpleasant imagery without trying to resolve it in any way.

FEEL EXERCISES TO DEAL WITH URGES AND THOUGHTS

Facing discomfort head-on is tough. You've had lots of experience doing the opposite— dodging, avoiding, or trying to drown it out. The urge to act is powerful. It's a well-practiced habit for you. And it's natural that old cut-and-run urges show up as you consciously choose to move into your discomfort with an eye on doing what you want to do in your life. Anxiety News Radio wants you to tune in 24/7.

It's important to be patient and kind to yourself. Breaking habits takes time. So far, you've been learning how to be with your anxious discomfort instead of fleeing, to soften instead of harden, to see beyond your critical mind and to connect with your values. Each time you practice these skills when you're anxious or afraid, you're rehearsing new behaviors that will, over time, become new habits. This will help you do more of what you care about when the old urges around anxiety and fear show up.

The next exercise, adapted from Hayes, Strosahl, and Wilson (2012), can be a real game-changer when you find yourself resisting urges and unwanted thoughts.

EXERCISE: Putting Thoughts and Urges on Cards

This exercise is your on-the-go tool for tackling WAF thoughts and urges. Grab some index cards or small pieces of paper. When those pesky WAFs show up, simply label them, placing each thought, worry, sensation, urge, or image on its own card. Use words to describe your WAFs.

After you've collected a short stack of these cards, take a close look at what you've written. If we asked you to describe what you see, what would you tell us? You're first reaction might be, "I see words...or a sentence." Or, maybe you see an emotion or a painful experience from your past. But here we want you to get more granular. What do you actually see on the card? Strip away the narrative. Focus on what's written as it is and not what your mind tells you is there.

If you take a moment and focus on what your eyes see, you'll eventually notice that you see words, letters, and ink. That's it. If you wrote down "I'm incompetent" and look, you'll see words, letters, and ink. Same for thoughts and urges like "I'm stupid," "I can't handle this," "Something bad will happen if I don't check," or "I have to get out of here." If you wrote "I am a banana," you'll see the same thing—words, letters, and ink.

All these thoughts are just ink on paper. They have no material form or substance. A moment ago the thoughts and urges were inside your head and probably felt like an enormous burden. Now, they're out in the open, exposed, and you can look at them. See them for what they are— just words, letters, and ink. Feel the weight lift as you acknowledge what they really are.

Here, it's important to ask yourself what happens when you turn your life over to the words, letters, and ink on each card. Do you do more or do less? Do you feel better or worse?

Notice that you have a choice to do what the card says, or you can allow what you wrote to be just as it is...words, letters, and ink expressing a thought...a sensation...an image...an urge to act.

You can also choose to struggle with what's on each card or to let it be if it's not helpful to you. To get a sense of the struggle, hold a card between your hands and push hard with each hand against the other for thirty seconds. Feel the resistance and discomfort while you're doing that. Then, let the card rest on your lap. Notice the difference between pushing against your thoughts and letting them be.

Carry these cards with you—in your pocket, bag, purse, or briefcase. Let them accompany you through the day. This will teach you that you can move with whatever arises within you. Occasionally glance at the cards, but don't get caught up in their message. Look and observe. It's just words, letters, and ink on paper.

Be mindful that you always have a choice to engage with what's on the cards or with something else in your life. Here, trust your experience, not your mind.

Make putting thoughts on cards a daily practice. Some people we've worked with tell us that they prepare a stack of index cards. Then, every morning, they shuffle them and pick four or five different cards to take along for the day.

Each time you touch or read a card without getting entangled, or doing what the card says, you're strengthening your resolve and freedom. The cards are there whenever you wish to attend to them, just like your old history is always with you.

The next exercise will give you more practice being with your WAF urges and not doing what they ask you to do. This exercise can be helpful anytime the urge to leave or avoid WAFs shows up.

EXERCISE: Stand Silently with Urges

In moments when old urges and impulses show up, remember you have choices. Keep it simple: in the heat of the moment, do nothing. Practice patience. Be still with your experience. Here's how:

Say and do nothing.

This suggestion is very much about staying with yourself instead of trying to avoid or run. You decide that you're not going to do what your mind and body are urging you to do, because it hurts you and your life. This choice may seem ridiculous and as unnatural as pushing into the finger trap. You can stop, be still, and wait until the stirring, raucous, and searing energy gradually softens and drifts away. You aren't suppressing anything here. You're just being honest with the fact that you're uncomfortable or hurt or sad or lonely or fearful, or whatever you're experiencing at the moment. And you stay with it, without feeding it or reacting to it. This will give you time to think about what you really want to be about in that moment and what you want to do moving forward.

Watch your mind machine.

We guarantee that the mind machine will be in overdrive doing its old thing. Don't get tangled up in what it's doing. Don't respond to it either. Just watch what it's doing from the compassionate observer perspective and meet that stirring energy with gentle acceptance. You don't need to get hooked. What you're experiencing is a part of you, but you the observer are so much more than that. Here, you're applying the skills of noticing each part of your experience as it is, and noticing that you can just notice without doing what you've always done in the past. This will give you space to consider other more vital options.

Ride the wild WAF horse.

This one is really tough. Sitting with discomfort and doing nothing while you feel like exploding or running is like trying to ride a wild horse. It can be very frightening. In that moment, bring attention to the physical experience of anxiety. Is there pressure? Is there tightness or contraction? Where, specifically, do you feel it? Does it have a shape? Here, perhaps for the first time, you can make a choice to sit and stay with the raucous energy and not do what you've always done. Try this out in your daily life. Once you are still, you can bring compassion and curiosity to the energy and pain. Look deeply into your experience without attempting to resolve it, fight it, or suppress it, and without acting on it. As you look, see if you can find the pain. Once you locate the pain, as in the previous exercises, look more deeply into it. Breathe into it, and then let it be.

Do the opposite.

This suggestion is inside all of the other suggestions we've made so far. Here, you decide to do the opposite of what your urges and impulses are pushing you to do. So, if you feel like avoiding, approach. Instead of lashing out, sit quietly. Pause and sit with the energy with kindness and self-compassion. Stay when your mind says to leave. Substitute checking or repeating actions with something aligned with your values. You can also create a list of urges and reactions, then jot down opposing actions. You could even put "do the opposite" on an index card or sticky note and carry it around as a reminder. This will help prepare you to do something new in the heat of the moment. You might also find it useful to visualize yourself doing the opposite with WAF-related urges and impulses. Mental rehearsal can help make new behaviors more likely.

Acting on WAF urges promises short-term relief but comes with lasting costs. It never solves the problem. Doing the opposite, even doing nothing and patiently embracing your experiences, can offer profound relief, relaxation, and connection with your inner softness and humanity.

In the next exercise you'll get to use your imagination. It's another opportunity to create space between your judgmental mind and your experience. If you can, listen to the audio first to enjoy the beautiful imagery.

EXERCISE: Leaves on a Stream

Start by getting centered and focus on the breath as you've done before. Just notice the gentle rising and falling of your breath in your chest and belly. There's no need to control your breathing in any way—simply let the breath breathe itself. Allow your eyes to close gently.

Then, after a few moments, imagine that you're sitting next to a small stream on a warm autumn day. As you gaze at the stream, you notice several large leaves of all colors, shapes, and sizes drifting along, each at its own pace, one by one, in the slowly moving current. Allow yourself to simply be there for a moment, watching.

When you're ready, gradually bring your awareness to what's going on inside you. As you do, gently notice and label each experience that shows up—thoughts, feelings, sensations, desires, and impulses. Perhaps one of those thoughts is *I don't have time for this.*

As the thoughts, feelings, sensations, desires, or impulses come along into your mind, notice them and gently place them one by one on each large leaf passing by. Observe as each leaf comes closer to you. Then watch as it slowly moves away, drifting along as it carries the contents of your mind and body out of sight downstream. Return to gazing at the stream, waiting for the next leaf to float by. Continue placing each thought, feeling, memory, or impulse on its own large leaf. Watch each one as you let them just float away downstream.

When you're ready, widen your attention to take in the sounds around you. Open your eyes and make the intention to bring gentle allowing and self-acceptance into the rest of your day.

Practice the Leaves on a Stream exercise every other day for a couple of weeks. As you improve, try it during real-life experiences with eyes open. Adopt the perspective of the stream, and from that perspective, hold each leaf (thought, feeling, sensation) and watch as it floats by without interference. Notice how you're becoming an observer.

LIFE-ENHANCEMENT EXERCISES

For the next two weeks, prioritize these self-care activities, aligning them with your values and life goals:

- See if you can catch when your personified WAF character shows up, and remind yourself that you don't have to listen.

- Practice the Kindly Allowing Anxiety exercise (from chapter 13) daily, with or without the audio.

- Use the FEEL Thought and Imagery Worksheet to track your progress with all the FEEL exercises in this chapter.

- Put WAF thoughts on cards and carry them with you.

- Cultivate mindfulness, observation skills, and kindness when anxiety arises. Just do the best you can.

THE TAKE-HOME MESSAGE

Developing comfort with your judgmental mind is one of the most powerful ways to end your WAF suffering. The exercises in this chapter and the entire book show that your WAF thoughts are like flies on barbless hooks—you can choose to let go, even if you've been tricked into biting. When you learn to disengage from your WAF thoughts and take them less seriously, they will no longer have the power to control you. The take-home message here is that if you stop struggling, you can get off the hook. This will give you freedom to swim toward your values.

My Mind Is Not My Enemy

Reflections:

- My mind is constantly generating thoughts—many are designed to help me. And I am grateful for that help.

- Although my mind is not my enemy, it's not always my best friend either. I don't need to trust, believe, or buy into everything my mind tells me, especially if it's unhelpful.

Inquiries:

- Am I willing to face my painful thoughts, memories, judgments, and urges as they are, so I can live the life I desire?

- Can I take the bold step to let go and bring compassion, kindness, and forgiveness to anxieties, fears, and other woundedness?

- Am I willing to make room for something radically new?

CHAPTER 15

Inhabiting Your Physical Body

When we come to that compassionate awareness that is not afraid of the fear, that can embrace the fear, we are able to heal the wounds of the child and the adult and begin to live the lives we've always wanted to live.

—Cheri Huber

As Cheri Huber teaches us in the opening quote, we must learn to embrace fear and cultivate self-compassion if we are to truly heal and live more fulfilling lives. There's no healthy way to bypass this process. In fact, trying to avoid this truth is what often keeps people stuck.

Here, you might be thinking, *Oh no—they're going to ask me to face my fears.* In a way, this is true, but this isn't about white-knuckling your way through your discomfort for its own sake or about proving something to yourself. This chapter is bigger than that. Building on the work you did in chapter 14, this chapter is about facing your life—and what you care about—while staying with your physical discomfort and bringing compassion to that experience. This is probably the kindest thing you can do for yourself.

And you won't be doing this naked, without any tools. You've been working on the skills you need to transform your anxiety and bodily discomfort into something you can have and let be, no longer resisting your experience.

The exercises in this chapter offer more opportunities to practice flexibility and softness with unpleasant sensations that keep you stuck. Like athletes stretching to maintain flexibility and prevent injury, life calls for flexibility too. Tightening around pain risks injury to your most precious commodity—your life.

GETTING WITH YOUR PAIN, LIVING YOUR LIFE

Pain is part of living fully. When you shut down to pain, you shut down to life. When you open up to life, you must open up to pain in all its forms. This is how it works. To have it all, you must be willing to have it all—the good, unpleasant, and sometimes ugly.

We're pretty certain that your WAF bodily discomfort is linked with what you care about—living out your values. In fact, if you look closely, you'll see that as you step toward what you care about, you'll risk getting something you don't want to have—anxiety, fear, unpleasant bodily sensations, disappointment, and so on. These are the barriers we talked about earlier in the book, alongside the more critical barriers associated with struggle and avoidance.

The solution is simple: to move into your life, you need to let go of the urge to act on your WAF discomfort and instead move with your feelings and bodily sensations, just as they are. This can be difficult to do. The same is true of other worthwhile experiences in life that are potentially good for you. Reflect on that for a moment.

Think back to a skill you now have that was once challenging. For example, think about your journey from starting an exercise routine to mastering it, from picking up a musical instrument to playing a tune effortlessly, or reflect on the progression from wobbling on a bike to riding confidently, from swinging a bat to hitting a home run.

Consider the evolution from embarking on a career to excelling in it, from fumbling with car controls to driving smoothly. Then, explore the complexities of navigating your daily roles as a friend, teacher, partner, spouse, or parent—learning to love, share, care, give, and forgive along the way. These and other examples teach us that to move forward—to accomplish our goals and create a life worthy of our time—we must be willing to face pain and difficulty. There's no other way around it.

To truly learn and grow, you must be willing to break free from any attachments to avoiding pain and seeking comfort. This cycle breeds unhappiness. The solution? Embrace discomfort while being connected to the moment-to-moment process of living your values.

For instance, you've probably heard people suggest that you should practice breathing in peace and relaxation and breathing out anxiety and tension. But this is more of the same, isn't it? You're grasping for what you desire with each inhale, and pushing away what you don't want on each exhale. What we're suggesting is the exact opposite of that. You decide to inhale the discomfort you're feeling anyway and exhale desires for what you want or think will bring relief. Here again, you're doing the opposite of what you typically do when WAFs show up.

If you let the words go—drop the unhelpful story line—and just feel the discomfort and sit with it without getting tangled up with it, you share what we all share. That's what compassion really means. Experiencing this sense of shared humanity has tremendous healing power—as Pema Chödrön (2001) tells us, it's the path out of misery and into vitality.

Breathing in pain and breathing out relief is the basis of an ancient form of meditation known as tonglen (meaning "giving and receiving"). Welcoming your pain and giving away good may strike you as odd. It goes against the grain. This is precisely why it can be so powerful.

When you embrace what you don't like, you transform it. That transformation will release you from attachment to pleasure seeking, fear, and self-absorption, and it will nurture your capacity for love and compassion. The next exercise will help you develop this important skill. Again, start by listening to the audio recording first at http://www.newharbinger.com/54476.

EXERCISE: Welcoming Discomfort, Giving Away Goodwill

Find a quiet spot where you won't be interrupted for five to ten minutes. Sit comfortably, whether on the floor or in a chair, with your palms facing up or down on your lap. If you wish, you may lie down on the floor with your hands resting at your sides.

When you're ready, close your eyes and focus on your breath's natural rhythm in your chest and belly. After a few moments, bring to mind a recent painful or anxiety-inducing event. Recall this event as fully as you can.

With your next inhale, visualize drawing in all the negativity and discomfort linked to the event, filling your lungs. As you do, acknowledge that what you're experiencing and inhaling is shared by millions of people worldwide. You're not alone in this; anxiety and other forms of pain and discomfort have been felt by countless people since the dawn of time.

Then, on each exhale, breathe out the wish for you and others to experience relief, joyfulness, peace, and goodwill. Imagine that your out-breath is illuminated in radiate white healing light, surrounding you and extending out to others in infinite ways. Do it slowly with the natural rhythm of your breathing.

Your intention here, for yourself and others, is for you and them to be free of any suffering, struggle, blame, and shame associated with the pain that you and they experience.

As you continue to breathe in, stay connected with your discomfort. With each exhale, send out goodwill and a heartfelt wish for others to find freedom from needless suffering.

If breathing in anxiety feels overwhelming, visualize breathing into a vast space or imagine your heart expanding infinitely with each inhale. Envision each in-breath enlarging your heart, creating enough space for all worries, anxieties, and concerns.

With each exhale, open yourself completely, embracing whatever arises without needing to push it away. You may experiment with imagining the in-breath as dark, murky smoke, and the out-breath as radiate bright healing light.

When your mind wanders or distractions arise, simply notice them kindly and return your focus to welcoming in your pain and releasing goodwill, kindness, and freedom from suffering on the out-breath. Keep practicing this giving and receiving as long as you wish.

Then, when you feel ready, slowly widen your attention and gently open your eyes, with the intention to bring this skill of compassionate giving and receiving into your daily experiences.

In daily life, practice this form of tonglen whenever you feel anxious, afraid, or uncomfortable. Nobody will know that you're inhaling your difficulty and sending out healing goodwill. Just breathe normally as you practice throughout your day. As you do, remind yourself that other people feel this, too, and that you're not alone in this, which will ease any sense of isolation and burden linked with your WAFs.

As you witness and accept your WAF discomfort and hurt, you'll be moving with and through what may seem difficult. As you do that, you'll be making room for compassion, kindness, and forgiveness. Through this process, you will:

1. Develop honesty about your experience, acknowledging discomfort without engagement. You'll also begin to see that you're not alone but are connected with all human beings who do experience pain and have the capacity to suffer with their pain.

2. Cultivate the courage to sit with your discomfort, stopping the urge to flee. As you do this, you're honoring yourself and your genuinely felt experiences as they are. No more running.

3. Enhance your ability to observe your experience without judgment, freeing yourself from reactive behaviors. This stance will free you to let go and move forward in your life.

So, when your mind gives you *This is difficult* or *This is too much*, kindly recognize those thoughts as a signal that you're on the path of something new and potentially vital. To help you along, we'll give you lots of opportunities for practice in this chapter using more FEEL exercises—remember, Feeling Experiences Enriches Living—to help you cultivate a new relationship with your physical body and painful past.

FEEL EXERCISES FOR BODILY DISCOMFORT

FEEL exercises have one purpose only—to help you engage your life to the fullest—and are therefore a natural extension of the exercises you've done throughout this workbook. Here, you'll get a chance to practice being an observer of your WAF bodily sensations, just noticing and experiencing them as they are while meeting them with a quality of kindness and compassion. When you do that, you'll be neutralizing the urge to avoid, run, or fix what your body is doing. Instead, you'll have the room to focus on what you want to do, what you want to be about, and where you want to go. As you get better at feeling, your life will grow.

FEEL Steps for Discomfort, in a Nutshell

FEEL exercises for bodily discomfort expand on the FEEL exercises you did for thoughts in chapter 14. To get started, you'll need to flip your willingness switch fully on. Next, focus on your deeply held values—what do you want to do and where do you want to go. Living your values unshackled from WAFs is the point of all of this. Keeping your values in mind will help you respond differently to bodily discomfort that has hindered you from living your life. It will also give you the motivation to persist even when you feel uncomfortable. So, you'll want to have your Valued Directions Worksheet and Life Compass handy and look for places where bodily discomfort has stood between you and your valued intentions.

The next step with these exercises is to gently create bodily sensations that typically trigger distress and send you into a tailspin. As you do, you'll be practicing mindful acceptance and kind allowing with physical discomfort and without struggle and resistance. This will change the way you respond to your discomfort.

In essence, these FEEL exercises entail choosing willingness, facing bodily discomfort with gentle kindness and allowing, and staying focused on your values. You'll have opportunities to create and watch bodily discomfort show up and then practice letting that discomfort be as it is. As you do that, you'll transform old discomfort difficulty into new discomfort vitality.

Practice and Pacing

All of the exercises require practice, practice, practice. You'll be familiar with the discomfort, but what you may not know is this discomfort without the added layer of struggle and avoidance. This new learning will take time.

So, take it slow. Don't rush through the exercises. It's best to repeat them several times in one sitting and then again over several days. Practice at home first. Find a place in your home to do the practice and make it a kind healing space. As you develop the skills, you can start applying them in your daily life. Let willingness, compassion, and values be your guide.

It's natural for your willingness switch to waver during the exercises, especially at the beginning. What matters is recognizing this and being willing to continue next time. Once you can keep your willingness switch on consistently, you're ready to progress to the next exercise.

A Word of Caution

You should expect some discomfort during the exercises. After all, you're willingly approaching what you typically avoid. You should also anticipate that your old history will show up right in your face, urging you to stop, struggle, or withdraw. The results of many research studies show that sticking with the program despite these urges can bring relief.

This relief may manifest as peace, reduced anxiety, or a sense that a burden has lifted. While discomfort may still arise occasionally, it will lose its intensity and power when you stop fighting it.

It's natural for you to want to feel better, but don't do the FEEL exercises chasing emotional outcomes—like feeling less anxious, keeping panic at bay, or stopping your mind from doing its thing—as this is just more of the same stuff that has never worked. The quality of your anxiety will likely change, but paradoxically this is most likely to happen when you don't chase emotional outcomes, like feeling better. Instead, focus on getting better at allowing your feelings, so you can move with them and do what you care about.

The goal of these FEEL exercises is to help you develop comfort and kindness in your own skin—to take the stance of being the chessboard or vessel and not the stuff you've collected as part of your learning history. This shift in perspective will free you up to live better with whatever your body and mind may be doing.

By shifting your perspective, anxiety will take a backseat, because you'll be spending less time with your WAF discomfort and more time focused on and engaging your life with your discomfort. That's how it works. That's how you get your life back. And that's the path to thinking and feeling better too. You can't experience peace so long as you remain in a fight with your mind and body.

Use this worksheet to track your progress with the exercises in this chapter. It can be downloaded at http://www.newharbinger.com/54476.

FEEL* Bodily Discomfort Worksheet

Instructions: Write down the date and time after completing the exercise, and record your reactions under each category.

Date: _____   Time: _____ a.m./p.m.

0	1	2	3	4	5	6	7	8	9	10
Low					Moderate					Extreme

Exercise	Sensation Intensity (Rate 0–10)	Anxiety Level (Rate 0–10)	Willingness to Experience (Yes or No?)	Struggle with Experience (Rate 0–10)	Avoidance of Experience (0–10)
Staring at a Spot	_____	_____	_____	_____	_____
Spinning	_____	_____	_____	_____	_____
Head Between Legs	_____	_____	_____	_____	_____
Shaking Head	_____	_____	_____	_____	_____
Breath Holding	_____	_____	_____	_____	_____
Breathing Through Straw	_____	_____	_____	_____	_____
Fast Breathing	_____	_____	_____	_____	_____
Fast Walking	_____	_____	_____	_____	_____
Jogging in Place	_____	_____	_____	_____	_____
Climbing Steps	_____	_____	_____	_____	_____
Other Aerobic Exercise	_____	_____	_____	_____	_____
Staring at Self in Mirror	_____	_____	_____	_____	_____

* Feeling Experience Enriches Living

How to Do FEEL Exercises in Eight Simple Steps

All of the FEEL exercises follow the same format. You'll want to have a watch or clock nearby. Remember to apply the skills you've been developing as you do each exercise. Here are the steps:

1. Identify a valued domain. Write down one important value on an index card or small piece of paper. Connect with this value before each practice session and keep it in mind as you do the exercises. Later, you can switch to another valued domain and repeat each FEEL exercise with your valued intentions in mind for that area.

2. Choose willingness. Are you willing to do each exercise to see what it's like to feel what you feel and think what you think when you're anxious or afraid? Be sure the answer is yes before moving on; otherwise, circle back to exercises covered earlier.

3. Practice a FEEL exercise. Begin the exercise and continue for thirty to sixty seconds past discomfort sensations or five minutes beyond the point when you first notice disturbing thoughts or images.

4. Apply mindful acceptance skills. Observe sensations, one at a time, with mindful acceptance and kindness for one to two minutes after stopping each exercise. Make space for your experiences.

5. Chart progress. Fill out the FEEL Bodily Discomfort Worksheet after each exercise to record your reactions and progress.

6. Reflect on practice. Take time to reflect on the practice you just did. Look at your ratings. Notice any unwillingness, struggle, or avoidance during the exercise. If you noticed any, try repeating the exercise more slowly. As you do, watch for sticky judgmental thoughts, such as *This isn't working* or *I can't stand this anxiety anymore*. See if you can notice these thoughts and make space from them from an observer perspective. You can also say to yourself, *I am having the thought that this isn't working*, or *My mind is feeding me the thought that I can't stand this anxiety anymore*, or *I'm having the thought that this is too much*. You can also label any thoughts as thinking.

7. Repeat FEEL exercises. Practice regularly, aiming for two to three repetitions per session. Allow mindful rest periods between exercises where you can sit comfortably and just notice your thoughts and sensations as they are.

8. Review ratings on the FEEL Bodily Discomfort Worksheet. You'll be ready to move on to a new exercise when your willingness rating is a consistent yes and struggle/avoidance levels are 3 or lower. Use your ratings as benchmarks for progress.

You can download a copy of the eight FEEL steps at http://www.newharbinger.com/54476. Keep these steps handy as you first do the exercises, and commit them to memory.

Physical Health Check

Before starting the exercises, ensure you are physically able to do them by consulting your doctor. Most involve mild-to-moderate physical activity. If you have been diagnosed with any of the following health conditions, we strongly suggest that you not do the FEEL exercises in this chapter until you've talked with your doctor.

- Asthma or lung problems

- Epilepsy

- A heart condition

- Physical injuries (neck, joint, back)

- Pregnancy

- History of fainting/low blood pressure

Should your doctor recommend against you doing one or more of these exercises, you can still practice the ones that have been approved for you. If your doctor recommends against all of these exercises, you can still practice applying your mindfulness skills and taking the observer perspective when you experience intense physical sensations as part of your regular daily activities. Remember that the goal is to practice staying with discomfort in all its forms without getting tangled up in it, whenever and in whatever form the discomfort may take.

EXERCISES: Being Willingly Dizzy

This set of exercises will help you practice mindful acceptance with sensations like dizziness, unsteadiness, or vertigo. The experience of dizziness will be different for everyone. It's an experience that occurs when you move your head and body through space at a rate too fast for your brain's balance system to keep up with.

Some people experience light-headedness, a sense of imbalance or floating, and nausea. These are all expected reactions. Here's how you can create them yourself:

- Staring at a spot. Position yourself about one to two feet from a nearby wall. Find a small spot on the wall and stare at it for about two minutes. Try to resist blinking as much as you can. Then, turn away quickly and focus on something else in the distance.

- Spinning. Using a swivel chair, spin yourself around as quickly as you can by pushing off of the floor as often as needed. Do this with your eyes open. You can then vary this by spinning your body while standing up with arms outstretched.

- Head between legs. Get in a sitting position. Place your head between your legs (at the knees) and hold that position for about thirty seconds. Then sit upright quickly. Do this gently if you have a history of back problems. You can play with this exercise by repeating it from a standing position.

- Shaking head. From a standing position, move your head back and forth and from side to side, slowly, with your eyes open. Do that for at least thirty seconds or until the sensations of dizziness are first noticed. Again, do this in a way that is steady and not too vigorous. Then stop and focus straight ahead.

To start these exercises, get set up in your healing space where you won't be disturbed, and have a clock or watch nearby. Be sure to position yourself in a spot where you won't fall or hurt yourself during the practice. Choose a dizziness activity and follow FEEL steps 1 to 8. Stay with and repeat the activity until you can tolerate discomfort without needing to stop (willingness rating yes, struggle/avoidance levels at 3 or lower). Then, move on to the next dizziness exercise and so on.

It's best to keep your eyes open as you do the exercises. It's fine if you need to sit down between practice sessions. Just watch that you don't immediately go to sitting or lying flat on the floor as a default coping strategy. If you can remain in a standing or sitting position while dizzy, you'll notice that the sensations will pass without you having to do anything about them.

Being willingly dizzy may have been hard for you. The experience can readily make anyone feel like they're losing touch with reality. The experience is not harmful to you, and the discomfort does pass. Congratulate yourself for practicing a new response to it.

EXERCISES: Being Willingly Out of Breath

The exercises in this section help you to make room for discomfort associated with breathlessness, heart sensations such as flutters, and chest tightness. These sensations, including dizziness and light-headedness and a sense of detachment from yourself, are common reactions. They're a natural byproduct of our normal blood-gas balance getting out of sync, specifically the balance of oxygen and carbon dioxide. Your body is set up to restore this blood-gas balance without effort on your part.

You can willingly bring on these sensations with any of the FEEL exercises below:

- Breath holding. For this exercise, simply take a deep breath and hold it for as long as you can. Start by doing the exercise while sitting down with your eyes open. You can then vary it by doing it longer the next time, while sitting, and then standing with eyes open or closed. Play with it. Be willingly creative with your discomfort.

- Breathing through a straw. For this FEEL exercise, use a straw and pinch your nostrils closed with your free hand while breathing through the straw. Aim for at least thirty seconds initially and gradually increase the duration. Experiment with different variations like closing your eyes or standing. The key is to proceed slowly and increase the challenge gradually as you learn to be with your discomfort without withdrawing.

- Fast breathing. Just about everyone has had the experience of being out of breath. When you breathe too quickly or too deeply, you take in too much oxygen relative to the carbon dioxide in your body. The technical label for this is hyperventilation. Though you may experience this response as beyond your control, you can bring it on by taking rapid inhales and exhales at a pace of about one breath every two seconds. When you first do this exercise, start in a sitting position. Take in a deep breath and then rapidly exhale fully, and repeat. Use a watch with a second hand and see if you can do it for at least sixty seconds at first and then work your way up to two or three minutes. This exercise is a powerful way to create a host of uncomfortable sensations that can keep you stuck and offtrack. And it is a great way to practice a new, more mindful response to them.

Take a moment to reflect on your practice and progress using the FEEL Bodily Discomfort Worksheet. Are you consciously choosing to keep your willingness switch on? Are you responding to discomfort with a softer, less engaged approach? Were you able to keep your values in focus during the exercises? Be patient and kind with yourself as you review your progress. It's okay if this doesn't come easily. And there's no need to rush. These small steps will lead to meaningful change in your life.

EXERCISES: Being Willingly Aerobic

Engaging your life requires action in the form of aerobic activity. If you've avoided activities, including exercise, because of the potential for WAF discomfort, then it's time to practice willingness by deliberately feeling the physical arousal that must happen within your body as you get moving. You'll see that there are many ways you can do that, and most have the added benefit of being good for your health. Here are a few:

- Fast walking. Walking engages your entire body. You can do this exercise indoors or outside. Start slow and work up to a fast and comfortable pace. Allow enough walking time so that you're able to notice and experience bodily WAF discomfort. It's best to do this exercise without other distractions (such as listening to music). When you can willingly be with your body while walking, you can then add the headphones.

- Jogging in place. This will give your heart rate and respiratory system a boost. And it can be practiced in your healing space at home. Refer to FEEL steps 1 to 8 as a guide.

- Climbing steps. Repeat going up and down a few steps until you begin to notice bodily discomfort. You can then increase the number of steps and duration of practice (such as two steps, five steps, ten steps, a flight or several flights of stairs).

- Other aerobic exercises. The possibilities for aerobic FEEL exercises are endless and could involve anything that gets your body going. Whether it's vacuuming, gardening, swimming, hiking, running errands, or even sexual activity, just follow FEEL steps 1 to 8 as you play with the possibilities.

Engaging in aerobic FEEL exercises not only gets you moving but also offers multiple benefits. These exercises provide a renewed sense of freedom, boost vitality, and expand your range of options. Throughout these exercises, remember to keep your values in mind—they're the whole point of why you're doing these exercises in the first place.

EXERCISE: Staring at Self in Mirror

This body scan exercise is about learning to be willingly present with yourself. Most of us don't like what we see when we look at ourselves in the mirror. There's always something about our bodies that could be different or better. The same is true of our sense of who we are—the part of us that is more than our hands, eyes, breasts, hips, or feet. It can be uncomfortable to see yourself exposed. Learning to be with yourself, just as you are, involves embracing your vulnerabilities and imperfections. This skill is particularly important in your interactions with other people.

This exercise involves looking at yourself in front of a full-length mirror for two to five minutes. The exercise is more powerful if you can do it undressed and fully exposed. Just like the earlier exercises, it will probably bring up some things that are uncomfortable.

Start by standing fully naked in front of a mirror so that you can see your entire body. Take a moment to look at yourself, really look. What do you see? What's it like to stand with yourself, unmasked, just as you are? Just notice any sensations coming from your body. See yourself from a kind perspective—there's nothing to be fixed, no need to hide anything. You are you.

Then shift your attention to your head and face. Notice the top of your head—your hair and skin. What does it really look like? Study it, noticing the textures, shape, and colors. Then gradually move to your face—eyes, nose, mouth, and cheeks. See if you can look closely into the natural beauty of your eyes—the colors, depth, and textures. Are those eyes something to be disliked or hated? What do you want to do with your seeing eyes, hearing ears, or your lips and mouth? See if you can allow yourself to be with your experience and let your mind do its own thing.

Then gradually move your attention to the area just below your chin. Slowly scan the midsection of your body—inside and out. What do you see as you gently focus on your shoulders, chest, belly, and each arm and hand? What do these parts of your body look like? Notice colors, textures, shapes, contours, and sensations from this region of your body.

Each part of your body is a part of you and has its own story to tell. What is your mind telling you about them now? Perhaps there is regret, shame, embarrassment, humiliation, or thoughts such as too big, too small, ugly, beautiful, wrinkled, smooth, attractive, or unattractive. What are you experiencing on the inside? Can you be with your body and mind just as they are—just as you are? Must you hide from yourself? Allow yourself time to just notice the labels your mind may be giving you, and then see if you can focus back on the raw, unedited experience of you.

Continue your body scan slowly, as you move your attention down to your feet and toes. Notice any inner discomfort that may show up. See if you can be with your discomfort as you spend this time with you. Is there anything about you that must be fixed?

Allow yourself to be with you just as you are—whole...complete...unique...perfectly imperfect...and vulnerable...like everyone else.

WHEN FEELING BODILY DISCOMFORT GETS TOUGH

This section is for times when you find yourself experiencing high levels of unwillingness, struggle, or the urge to avoid or stop your practice. This isn't a time to cave in to what your mind might be feeding you. What you need to do here is to do your practice more slowly and with greater simplicity of focus. So instead of being with the entire experience, bring your kind attention to two or three bodily sensations, one at a time.

EXERCISE: Staying with Intense Bodily Discomfort

Choose one challenging bodily sensation to focus on. Acknowledge its presence by simply stating what you're experiencing: I am noticing tension, I am noticing fast breathing, I am noticing my heart beating, or I am noticing dizziness, light-headedness, or the sensation of heat or the sensation of cold.

Acknowledge any discomfort, stay with it, breathe through it, and approach it with kindness. Just like in the finger trap and Kindly Allowing Anxiety exercises, this is an opportunity to welcome the discomfort instead of resisting or avoiding it.

If you need to, you can slow the process. To do that, close your eyes for a moment, allowing _____ (insert the uncomfortable sensation) to be what it is, a feeling in your body, nothing more and nothing less.

Then, ask yourself, *Where else have I felt this sensation?* Maybe it was while mowing the lawn or on a hot day outdoors. Perhaps during a pleasant surprise or in an everyday activity. Acknowledge that you've felt this bodily sensation before, then proceed to other inquiries:

- Do I need to resist this sensation, or can I accept its presence and allow space for it?

- What does this sensation really feel like? Where does it start and where does it end?

- Is this sensation my enemy, or can I have it as a feeling, a sensation?

- Is this sensation something I must not or cannot have? Even if my mind tells me that I can't have it, am I willing to create space for it in my heart?

- Must I fight against this sensation, or is there room within me to acknowledge and experience it just as it is? Can I cultivate kindness toward myself in this moment?

As you make space for each sensation, one by one, you may notice that your mind is feeding you all sorts of labels—old F-E-A-R (False Evaluations Appearing Real) labels—like *This is dangerous, It's getting worse, I can't deal with it*, or *I'm losing control.* When that happens, simply thank your mind for such labels. Then gently shift your attention back to watching and noticing with gentle curiosity, openness, and compassion.

This exercise strengthens your ability to direct your attention and choose a softer approach to discomfort, regardless of whether you like what you're feeling. Remember, it's okay not to like feeling uncomfortable as long as you're willing to feel what you feel.

You can shift your mindset by applying mindfulness strategies and exercises from previous chapters to help you move with physical discomfort. For instance, transform *I want to get better but...it's very hard* into a more honest and correct statement, like *I want to get better, and I'm having the thought this is very hard*. Remember, you control how you relate to the sensations your body creates.

LIFE-ENHANCEMENT EXERCISES

For the next two weeks, prioritize these activities on your to-do list:

- Practice tonglen and the FEEL exercises for bodily discomfort. If possible, do some every day and record your progress.

- Do the Kindly Allowing Anxiety exercise (chapter 13) once a day, and don't leave out your favorite loving-kindness and self-compassion practices.

- Continue to practice the I Am meditation at least once a day. It will help you be the silent observer of your experience (the chessboard) rather than a struggling player with an agenda.

- Apply mindfulness skills and take an observer perspective during daily activities.

- Decide to do something, however small, in line with your values and do it with your willingness switch turned on.

THE TAKE-HOME MESSAGE

Facing discomfort with kindness and willingness is the first step out of anxious suffering and toward a more vibrant life. Choose to nurture this skill through practice, and then work to apply it wherever you find yourself. By embracing discomfort as it is—rather than running away from it—you free yourself from its grip. Situations or triggers that evoke discomfort—many of them linked with your values—will be less likely to derail you. Being open and willing to feel what you feel and think what you think is how you'll reclaim your life. Actively engage with the exercises instead of waiting for change to come to you. Practice and experiment with them. Be the resolute driver of your Life Bus.

Facing Discomfort for My Growth and Liberation

Reflections:

- It's tempting to avoid bodily discomfort, but true strength lies in facing it openly, honestly, and with compassion. At its root, discomfort is pain—physical, mental, emotional.

- The mind creates the illusion that you can't feel this, but you can. Embracing discomfort with kindness leads to new possibilities and freedom from fear.

Inquiries:

- Am I willing to acknowledge and experience unpleasant bodily sensations and not let them stand between me and what I want to do?

- Must these sensations really be my enemy?

- Am I willing to face my discomfort as it is, accepting myself with all my flaws, weaknesses, and vulnerabilities?

CHAPTER 16

Making Peace with the Past

Even though you may want to move forward in your life, you may have one foot on the brakes. In order to be free, we must learn how to let go. Release the hurt. Release the fear. Refuse to entertain your old pain. The energy it takes to hang onto the past is holding you back from a new life. What is it you could let go of today?

—Mary Manin Morrissey

You have a past. Everyone does. It's full of moments—dark, bright, and neutral. Most of us remember very little of it. Still, you know there's much more to your past than that small bit you can remember. What you remember can leave you feeling more alive or torn apart and wounded.

Your response to these memories determines their impact on your life. Maybe it's time to let go of remnants from the past that no longer serve you.

All moments of your past are in the vessel that you call you. But you are not the history you've had. You are not the experiences that ended up in your vessel. You are the holder and witnessing observer of your life—your own safe refuge. This distinction is important to understand, because it will help you make peace with your past.

You were there before the sweet and dark moments you lived through. You were there before the hurt you endured, the trauma you suffered, or even the mundane moments of your past. And you are here now, in this moment looking forward, with a life of possibility ahead of you.

Sometimes we get wisdom from remembering past trials and traumas we've endured, and we leverage that to live more wisely and fully now. You may discover an inner strength, a renewed appreciation for life, and an inner resolve not to repeat the hardships you endured. Often though, painful memories have the opposite effect. They keep us stuck in the past, reliving old wounds that do not serve us well from this point forward in our lives.

There are many ways to get stuck in the past. Maybe you've been trying to figure it out, make sense of it, or understand. Or, maybe you relive traumas you endured during combat or at the hands of someone else—a parent, a stranger, or a once-trusted friend or partner. You may remember and be overwhelmed by guilt and shame. Or, you may be attached to the good times, the way things once were, wishing you could have that again.

In these moments, we forget the simple truth that change is constant, time only moves forward, and nothing remains the same.

All this doesn't mean that you forget your past. You don't ignore the rearview mirror driving your car. But you don't fix your eyes on that mirror either, always looking back as you're trying to move forward. That would have disastrous consequences.

Rather, you acknowledge your past as the past—sometimes it's important to look in the rearview mirror at what's behind you. Then you decide to learn from it and refocus on the present while keeping your eyes and heart looking forward. This is the only way to get where you want to go in life.

The past cannot be changed. The future has yet to be. All we really have is the present. And it turns out that learning to be present is a powerful way to break free from the hooks and snares of your past. In fact, the present is the only place where you can do something to make a difference in your life. You've got to be in the driver's seat, right now, to guide your Life Bus forward.

We're going to help you learn to do this in a way that honors your past, however painful. In fact, the larger message of this chapter is about finding a way to make peace with your past—to simply allow it to be as it was, and not get drawn into the drama and pulled out of the present.

Before going forward with the next section, we'd like you to pause and center yourself as you've done so many times before. Remind yourself of why you're here and the important work you're doing to heal and reclaim your life.

EXERCISE: Your Past and You

Let's start with a simple exercise that will teach you something about how the mind works with memory. We're going to share two numbers. Don't write them down. Ready? The numbers are 4 and 3.

Now, respond to each of the following questions silently to yourself.

What were the numbers? Suppose we were to ask you ten minutes from now, do you think you could tell us the numbers? What about if we asked you at the end of this chapter?

Suppose we made it worthwhile to you, like, say you'd get a million dollars if you could tell us the numbers ten years from now. Do you think you could do it? We bet you could. What were the numbers again?

Let's step back and look at this. In mere seconds, we implanted a history in your mind that has now become a memory. Now, you have two random numbers, with no real significance, swirling around in your head.

Notice that you didn't choose to have those numbers in your head. We did. And now, they're etched into your consciousness, ready to be recalled at will.

This simple exercise teaches that you often have little control over what becomes a part of your history, your vessel, and eventually your memory. But you can control how you respond.

WHAT IS A MEMORY ANYWAY?

When you remember something, you're always doing it in the present moment. Painful memories are reminders of the past. That's it. They have no real substance. They're often entwined with internal experiences and can be readily triggered by external events.

Yet all memories are collections of images, thoughts, physical sensations, and emotions. These can show up in an instant. When they do, you often add to them based on your lived experiences since the remembered event. This is why what you remember often ends up distorted over time.

When you remember something painful, you may feel a range of unpleasant emotions. What you feel is real and a genuine aspect of your experience. But a painful memory is not the same as going through the hurtful or life-threatening event you endured. This can be hard to grasp.

If you step back, you'll see that the memory hurts and seems real, but there's nothing you can do now to undo it, change the outcome, or bring about any resolution. And there's nothing you need to do either. The event is in your past. You are in the present. This is what we mean when we say, "Painful memories are not the event." The only thing repeating now are thoughts and the emotional pain. What is not repeating is the actual event, although your mind works hard like an experienced Hollywood film director to make it as real as possible.

What Goes In, Stays In

Your painful past may resurface time and again. That's because we are all historical beings. Again, we all come into the world like an empty vessel, and very quickly we start to collect different kinds of experiences. Some of these you choose, and others happen outside your control.

This process of collecting experiences will continue for as long as you're alive. Nothing is subtracted or deleted. What goes in, stays in, short of brain insult or injury. Some of it you'll remember easily; other experiences not so much. But it's all in there.

You've seen that your mind and body are always producing thoughts and sensations that you have little control over. Memories are like that too—they can pop into your awareness without much effort. Here are a few examples.

Read the following words and fill in the blanks:

- Twinkle, twinkle, little _____.

- Little Miss Muffet sat on a _____.

If you grew up in the West, it probably took you seconds to fill in the blank with the first example. Because we share that history with you, we're confident you responded with "star!" Notice that thinking that word when you did was not a choice—it just showed up in your awareness with a few prompts.

Depending on your age, you may have struggled with knowing that "tuffet" is the correct answer to the second fill-in. But even if you didn't know the answer, you know now. So next time you're around someone who says, "Little Miss Muffet sat on a _____," you'll be able to respond boldly with "tuffet." Why? Because the word "tuffet" is now part of your history.

For those of you who knew the correct answer, we might ask you when was the last time you used the word "tuffet"? ("Hey, pull up a tuffet, and let's have some coffee.") You probably don't remember exactly when and where you learned that nursery rhyme, but it's in there and can be conjured up in seconds with the right prompts.

Memories also often come with vivid imagery, like scenes from a movie playing in your mind. Some are crystal clear, while others are vague impressions. Importantly, images are often tainted by the mind's endless judgments and interpretations, accompanied by a spectrum of sensations and emotions—some pleasant, others heavy and dark. They can be brought to mind just like the words "star" and "tuffet."

And you know what? Being able to remember can be a wonderful gift too. Even painful or traumatic experiences can be used wisely to help you move forward and avoid past mistakes.

Barbara, a stay-at-home mother of two, is a good example of what we mean. She told us that her upbringing was rough. She suffered neglect and verbal and physical abuse at the hands of her parents and sexual abuse from an uncle who lived next door. In describing her past, Barbara acknowledged the pain she endured. "No child should have to go through that," she said. Yet, she also shared this: "I went through hell as a kid, but you know what? Those experiences made me stronger and more resolved to never, ever repeat what I went through with my kids. I learned what not to do from my parents, and that solidified my desire to be the most supportive, loving, and caring parent that I can be to my two little ones. I'm not going to pass on the hurt I endured to my kids or anyone else, including myself."

Barbara went through a lot, but she wasn't willing to be a victim of the harsh treatment she endured long ago. When she remembered her childhood, she felt pain, and tears flowed at times. This response is exactly what we'd expect, given her past. She should feel something.

But Barbara was also determined not to repeat the abuse she endured with her kids. Some call this "post-traumatic growth," but whatever words are used, the point is to break free from the shackles of unhelpful memories associated with a painful past. Barbara decided to put her attention on her kids and the life she wished to create for them, including the mother she wished to be. She didn't forget her past. In fact, it motivated her to live her best life going forward.

Of course, this isn't ever easy to do, but it can be done with the skills you're learning and with the right mindset. What is that mindset?

Simply, it's being willing to acknowledge your painful past, learn from it, and let it go, so you can move forward, grow, and live your life. So long as you are tethered to the past, you won't be able to move forward. You have to decide, "I'm not doing that anymore…I'm not going to live my life as damaged, the victim, broken, hopeless."

Getting Hooked on Your Past

It's easy to get hooked on the past—be it cherished moments you cling to or painful memories you'd rather discard. Maybe it's combat, or it's an accident, or rape, loss, abuse, regrets, missed opportunities, or choices that you wish you could undo. It may be a difficult childhood, or anger and resentment at how your parents and friends treated you.

Recalling painful moments may evoke overwhelming guilt or shame, whereas good memories may evoke nostalgia. Yet, there's nothing inherently wrong with remembering both the bad and the good—it's how we learn and grow.

It's okay that you don't like remembering some of your past. Everyone has things they would rather forget. Some have worse things in their past than others do—but everyone has something. But getting stuck in the past is a trap you must avoid. The next exercise will show you why.

EXERCISE: Stuck Stirring a Bucket of Shit

Imagine that you're sitting next to a large bucket with a heavy wooden ladle. This bucket is your past. You try to resist opening the lid, but for whatever reason, the lid pops off. Now, you find yourself staring down into the bucket, only to find that it's full of shit and it really smells awful. Desperate to lessen the stench, you begin stirring, hoping in vain for a change.

In a way, fixating on the past is like stirring this foul concoction endlessly. Along with that, your mind echoes a stream of self-defeating messages—telling you that you're stuck, unworthy, broken, wrong, hopelessly damaged. And still, you sit and stir the pot, going back, reopening old wounds, regrets, painful experiences.

Maybe you think that if you stir the shit long enough, something will change. But truthfully, no amount of stirring can change it. If anything, it only exacerbates the stench and creates chaos, leaving you drained.

Here's something else to notice—all of this remembering, reliving, and stirring is happening now, in the present. This is important to notice. There's no time machine to revisit the past; time only moves forward, and so must you.

To break free from this cycle, you must stop stirring: acknowledge the past for what it is, drop the unhelpful narratives your mind conjures, and focus on the present moment. Then, you'll be able to focus on where you are, right now, what you want to do, right now, and how you can move toward what matters, right now.

By recognizing remembering for what it is—your mind thinking—you can approach it with gentle curiosity and kindness. That's how to free yourself from the grip of a painful past.

Importantly, this doesn't mean forgetting or condoning past wrongs or challenges you endured. Instead, you're being invited to learn from the past, open up to it because it's there anyway, and carry it forward in ways that dignify your life. So, if you're willing, let's get started.

DEFUSING FROM A DIFFICULT PAST

When a painful or traumatic memory pops into your awareness, it's easy to lose touch with the present moment. When this happens, pause, take slow deep breaths, and acknowledge what's happening. You're remembering, which is just another form of thinking. And notice that you're doing it now, from the safe refuge of the present moment.

We know that this can seem hard at first. If you struggle with painful thoughts about your past or feel disconnected from your body and surroundings—like you're in another place—then you know how challenging it can be to recover your sense of grounding. Being in that place is unsettling and makes it difficult to focus on what's important now.

So, if you're willing, let's do an exercise that will help you regain your ground when you've been snared by thoughts about your past. Just five minutes is all you need, and with practice, you'll master grounding yourself wherever you are. Again, we recommend that you listen to the audio recording at http://www.newharbinger.com/54476 and follow along.

EXERCISE: Grounding in the Now

Start by removing your shoes if you can, and get in a comfortable position, sitting upright and breathing naturally. Or, if you prefer, you can do this exercise standing, with knees slightly bent.

Once you're ready, close your eyes and bring your attention to your breath. Notice where you feel your breath most strongly. Perhaps it's in your chest, abdomen, or nostrils.

Now bring your attention to your feet. Feel them contacting the floor and ground beneath you. Notice the sense of pressure of your body against the earth below.

Go ahead and wiggle your toes for a moment, and then scrunch your feet into balls by curling your toes downward toward the ground. Notice the movement of the small bones of your feet, and the soft tissue between the bones. Allow yourself to bring all of your attention to these movements. And notice that you can notice them.

Next, bring your awareness to how your feet feel, and notice any sensations there, like tension, relaxation, pain, pressure, warmth or coolness, or even no sensation. Again, noticing that you can notice them.

Go ahead and gently press your feet into the ground beneath you. Become aware of feeling a strong contact with the ground. Then ease up, allowing your feet to contact the floor naturally.

Now, imagine that your breath is passing in and out through your feet as you take a deep, rich inhale...and then a slow exhale. On the next in-breath visualize the pores of the soles of your feet breathing in and filling your body with the solid foundational energy of the earth beneath you. On your out-breath, feel your feet discharging this energy back into the earth, creating strong roots.

Continue on like this—grounding to the earth and where you are now. Notice the dynamic connection between you and the earth and your surroundings. And, if you find your attention wandering, bring it back to your feet, deeply breathing in and out through them and feeling the grounding earth connection...

As this time for practice comes to a close, direct your attention back to the room. Notice the sounds in the room, the feeling of your body as you sit or stand, the temperature of the air, the position of your body, the smells in the room, the feeling of the air on your skin.

And notice that you're here in the now—present, alert, and alive. When you're ready, gently open your eyes and carry this grounding presence with you into the present moment and the rest of your day.

If you have an injury, then modify the practice by focusing on a part of your body that's in contact with any surface beneath you. Use the audio to guide you until you have mastered grounding. Then, do it on your own. Practice this exercise regularly, as it fosters seeking refuge in your own present awareness. This practice equips you to reclaim your ground when you find yourself being pulled into difficult memories.

You can also ground yourself by engaging your senses deeply: taste something strong like a lemon, smell pungent scents like soap, touch objects that have unusual texture, shape, or weight, look at something bright or unusual, or listen to sounds or music.

As you practice grounding, be mindful of your intentions—sensory engagement should serve to reconnect you with the present, so you can act of your values now. Don't use grounding to escape or avoid painful memories. That's just more of the same, and it doesn't work.

Experiment with these grounding techniques to find what works best for you.

THE MANY STORIES OF YOU

Your mind, much like a film director, crafts a narrative of your past, selectively choosing which scenes to include in the story line. Yet this narrative often overlooks important moments, both dark and light, creating an incomplete story. You know this if you struggle with traumatic memories. The narrative with trauma is often tragic and limiting.

To craft your whole narrative, you must be willing to explore the omitted moments of your past and consider alternative stories. This requires curiosity, openness, and a willingness to let go of the current narrative.

The next writing exercise will guide you through this process. All you need is willingness, curiosity, paper, and something to write with. Remember, this is about breaking free from the constraints of your past, honoring your history, and moving forward in alignment with your values. You'll need about fifteen minutes. Feel free to take more time with this exercise too.

EXERCISE: The Story of You

Begin by capturing the dominant narrative your mind constructs about your life. Picture yourself in a theater, watching your past unfold on a colossal screen. What experiences and events does your mind consistently emphasize? What moments define the story of you, according to your mind's script?

Your Life Movie—Take 1

Go ahead and write one paragraph describing the narrative that naturally emerges from your mind. Write freely without censoring yourself. It's okay if the story leans toward darker moments or if it encompasses a mix of experiences. Let it flow as if no one will ever read it—no editing, no holding back. When you're ready, continue reading.

Once you're done writing, pause and take a few slow breaths. Then read what you've written aloud, paying attention to the words, letters, and ink that depict your past and your identity. Observe the story unfolding before you, like the chessboard observing the game. What tone does the narrative take? How old does it feel? How does it grip and entangle you? Is there anything in the narrative that you absolutely cannot think about right now? Is there anything you're experiencing now that's really your enemy? Notice any resistance or discomfort that arises, and do your best to observe it with kindness and impartiality. Take your time with this process before continuing.

Your Life Movie—Take 2

Now, we want you to craft another script that keeps all factual events from Take 1—those experiences you've actually lived through. However, this time, you'll be adding to the story.

Consider what experiences might be missing or overlooked by your mind. What else could be added to enrich the narrative? Think of moments, big or small, that may have slipped under the radar or require a bit of effort to recall. Whether neutral, sweet, or dark, it doesn't matter—include them all. Also, don't worry about whether they align with the original story line; instead, focus on weaving in experiences from your history, no matter how insignificant they may seem—like eating a hamburger, taking a hot shower, or watching a movie.

Allow yourself at least five minutes to write and refine this narrative, aiming for a longer story than Take 1. Once you've captured it on paper, continue reading.

Once more, take a moment to pause and center yourself with a few slow, grounding breaths. Then, read aloud the narrative you've written, observing the words, letters, and ink on the page with kindness, curiosity, and gentleness. Reflect on the story that unfolds before you—how does it differ from the first? Does this more complete version evoke similar emotions and reactions to those evoked by Take 1? Notice in particular if there are elements of the story that you don't like to think about or experience right now. Then ask yourself, ***Must the stuff on the page really be my enemy, something that I cannot think about now?*** Reflect on these questions for a moment before continuing. Then, when you're ready, continue reading.

Your Life Movie—Take 3

Now, if you're willing, we'd like you to repeat this exercise at least one more time. This time keep the narrative from Take 2 and expand upon it with additional experiences you've had. Think as small or as large as you wish, allowing yourself to include both distant and recent experiences. Then, rewrite the script without removing anything, regardless of the size or significance of the events. This story should be longer than Take 2. Give yourself about five minutes to write. When you're done, continue reading.

Once more, take a moment to pause, allowing yourself to breathe deeply. Then, read aloud the narrative you've written, adopting the perspective of an observer.

Notice the words, letters, and ink on the page—observe them with kindness, curiosity, and gentleness. Consider the story that unfolds before you—how does it compare to the previous versions? Are there elements of the story that you don't like to think about or experience now? Also notice that ultimately all three takes are just stories—words, letters, and ink on a page.

Take a few moments to reflect on these questions before continuing. When you feel ready, move on and continue reading.

This exercise can be challenging at first, and that's okay. Go as far with this exercise as you're willing to go. Each time you rewrite and add to the story of you, you'll notice that there's more to you than the one-sided dark story that your mind usually gives you. The story of you will continue to be written for as long as you're alive. The trick is to observe all your experiences, looking for bits that your mind leaves out or ignores. You don't have to continue to buy into the one-sided dark drama about your past.

It's also important to look for things your mind adds that are not part of the facts of your past. For instance, suppose you were in a terrible car accident, and you were at fault. In your narrative, your mind may add things like *You're such an idiot… You'll never be able to drive again… You deserve to rot in hell… You can never forgive yourself.*

These judgments are not the facts but merely evaluations about your past and you. Watch for them and, if you like, edit your narratives to delete all evaluations and judgments about you, the event, and those involved. Stick with the facts that are true to your lived experience. In the example just given, the facts are that you were in a car accident and legal authorities determined you were at fault. That's it.

Importantly, look to see what's useful from your past in guiding your life from this point onward.

MAKING PEACE WITH YOUR PAST

In the upcoming exercises, you'll learn how to transform your relationship with your past—moving from one that's adversarial to one that's kind, gentle, and peaceful. You'll also discover how to release thoughts about the past that no longer serve you, as you cultivate a healing response to old wounds.

This may not be easy at first, but if you stick with it and practice a few times over this week, you may notice that your past loses some of its power to steer your Life Bus offtrack. You can heal yourself. You can learn to let go, without forgetting. You can carry your past forward and create the life you long to lead. The past can't stop you unless you let it.

Each exercise will take about fifteen minutes. We recommend starting with the guided audio at http://www.newharbinger.com/54476 and then progressing to independent practice once you're familiar with the exercises.

EXERCISE: Being Kind with Old Wounds

Begin by getting yourself in a comfortable position. Sit upright and allow yourself to get grounded with a few slow breaths in...and out, from the earth below you, up your torso, and then back out through the soles of your feet, rooting strongly in the earth below.

Now bring to mind a memory that you've been struggling with for a very long time. See if you can put yourself in that situation. Where were you? What happened? What were you doing? What were others saying or doing? Watch it as if it were unfolding on a giant movie screen. See if you can give yourself permission to be present with this experience as fully as you can. Notice how you reacted then. Also notice how you're reacting to the memory now.

Slow things down as best you can...and notice thoughts as thoughts, images as images, physical sensations as sensations, emotions as emotions...just as they are. Watch and gently observe parts of your experience as they come and go, as you take the perspective of the chessboard or vessel. There's nothing to do but notice. You don't have to take sides...just stay with this experience as best you can and breathe.

When you're ready, release that difficult image with a large grounding breath in and out through your feet, and then imagine an earlier time in your life—one long before the events that comprise your difficult memory.

Go back as far as you can remember...to a time in your childhood when you remember feeling good, even for a brief time. See if you can visualize that younger you—notice your face and eyes as a child, your hair, what you were wearing, and how small you were. How old is this younger version of yourself? Also notice where you were, what you were doing, what you were experiencing that left you feeling whole and complete, even if that good feeling was short-lived.

Now, imagine that younger you is standing in front of you now and then slowly walks over and sits on your lap. As you hold that younger you on your lap, you look into their little eyes and see that they're looking back at you. You then become aware that your younger you has no idea what the future holds. But you do. You know the truth of what's to come. You know what's coming because you've lived through it.

As you look into the eyes of your younger self, what advice would you share with them, knowing all that you know about what's coming in their future? How would you respond to that younger you? What does that little child need from you right now? What do they need to hear from you right now? Take a moment to express, with words or a gesture, what you'd like to share with your younger you. Say the words out loud. Notice also that you were there then, and you're here now too.

Linger with this experience for a few moments. Then, when you're ready, say good-bye to your younger self and wait until they have left the room. Then, allow yourself to come back to an awareness of sitting where you are right now...see if you can bring a sense of kindness to your experience now and to any old wounds that you remember. As you do, place your hands over your heart and give yourself the words you shared with the smaller you. Sense any gentleness and compassion you may have felt with the younger you and extend that to yourself and your experience now. What do you need right now?

Sit this way as long as you wish—just caring for yourself, being with yourself, giving yourself comfort, rest, healing, and support. Gently remind yourself that you're more than what you lived through, however difficult or painful it may be to remember.

Then, when you're ready, take a final grounding breath or two, and gently open your eyes—with or without tears, it doesn't matter. Simply allow yourself to come back to the present, with the intention to bring kindness to yourself, your history and old wounds, and your life.

This exercise can evoke strong emotions. You might feel moved to tears or experience a sense of numbing or resistance. You have had a hard time giving yourself the same compassion that you just gave to your younger self. Conversely, you might also feel a profound sense of peace, as if a weight has been lifted. Whatever your experience, it's valid and perfectly okay.

The essential insight is that you were there before the dark moments of your past, and you possess the power to transform your relationship with your past now. You can opt to approach your old memories in a kinder, peaceful, and more loving way. In fact, you have an abundant capacity to do just that. Nothing from your past can rob you of that without your consent.

The Power of Forgiveness

When people hear the word "forgiveness," they often jump to conclusions. You may too. Your mind may tell you that forgiveness means condoning or forgetting past wrongs or, worse, ignoring the hurt and pain you suffered at the hands of someone else or even pain that was self-inflicted. You may see it as a sign of weakness or as something that you must feel in your bones before you take steps to forgive. None of these are true.

When the late Pope John Paul II met to forgive his would-be assassin, he wasn't condoning the attempt on his life. Instead, he was extending mercy and compassion. He was letting go of the burden he was carrying of being the target of a senseless act. The assassin still sat in prison for his crime. This is the essence of forgiveness—it's nothing more than letting go of a painful past so that *you* can heal and move on!

> *Forgiving yourself and others is the only path to healing.*

You alone hold the power to forgive. You do it because clinging to past hurts traps you as a perpetual victim, longing for a resolution that may never arrive. Grudges poison your spirit, stifling happiness and growth. Refusing to forgive hurts you, and it does nothing to resolve past injustices or punish those who wronged you. This is why it needs to stop. It's time to let go.

Learning to forgive is the most powerful way to loosen the grip of your painful past. Studies show forgiveness improves physical, emotional, and spiritual health. Those who learn this important skill experience less hurt, stress, anger, depression, and illness. They also report experiencing a greater capacity for hope, optimism, compassion, love, and an abiding sense of well-being. These are the concrete benefits of forgiveness.

Beyond the benefits, letting go will give you the space to move forward with your life. Forgiveness frees you from old stories, shame, and pain, allowing you to chart a new path forward. It's a powerful choice that will help you create the life you want now.

Conversely, if you don't let go and forgive others for the harm they did, they and their deeds will continue to haunt you, harm you, and have a hold on you. Every moment you hang on to resentment, you hurt yourself one more time. You also destroy your peace of mind and give the past and any wrongdoers power over your life now. That is, by not forgiving, you only hurt yourself. Remember, this practice is for you, not for the people or the circumstances that once hurt you! It will help you heal emotional wounds and release the burdens of the past.

The next exercise outlines four steps to take on the path to choosing forgiveness as an act of letting go of past wrongs:

- **Step 1: Awareness**—facing hurt and pain as it is, without judgment or denial

- **Step 2: Separation**—using your observer self to soften and invite healing and change

- **Step 3: Compassionate witness**—extending compassion to your experience and others

- **Step 4: Letting go and moving on**—releasing grudges and resentment that fan the flames of your suffering, and then moving forward in your life in directions you want to go

EXERCISE: Learning to Let Go of Grudges

A grudge is a persistent feeling of ill will or resentment, typically stemming from a past insult or injury. Holding a grudge involves harboring anger or resentment toward someone for a perceived wrong or injustice, often without seeking resolution or forgiveness.

With this definition in mind, take a moment to reflect on a grudge you harbor. Consider a situation or an event that evokes feelings of anger, hurt, resentment, bitterness, or a desire for justice. Grab a piece of paper and meticulously document the specifics of the past transgression. Leave no detail unexamined.

When you're ready, close your eyes and bring the event to mind. Really get into it as best you can. What happened? Who wronged whom? How were you or others harmed? What didn't you get then that you're longing for now? Maybe it was safety and protection or respect and consideration. It could be love, support, loyalty, friendship, or something else. Spend a few minutes fully immersing yourself in this memory.

Acknowledge the pain associated with the event, as it is. Where do you feel it in your body? See if you can create space for all of it. What does the pain feel like? What does it look like?

Notice and observe your mind's tendency to judge, blame, and criticize. Try to adopt a detached perspective as a silent observer, separating the raw pain from your mind's evaluations of your pain. Notice judgment as judgment, blame as blame, and bitterness as bitterness, without engagement. Simply observe without getting entangled in these thoughts.

See if you can step back further, as if observing the event on a giant screen. Imagine being in the audience, witnessing the drama unfold with fresh eyes. Open your heart as a compassionate witness of all actors in this scene—who's causing harm, who's suffering—including you too. Recognize the person responsible for the pain, both then and now.

Now kindly ask yourself these questions: *Who's responsible for letting go now? Who controls whether resentment lingers or dissipates? Who suffers from holding on to past grievances? Who has the power release the grudge and move on?* The answer is *you*.

You can redirect the energy spent on resentment and put it toward the life you wish to live. You can bring kindness to your experience by facing your pain squarely for what it is. Own it because it is yours, and then choose to let it go—release it.

If letting go feels challenging, consider who truly suffers by holding on—is it you or the one who wronged you? Imagine the freedom and peace that come with releasing the grudge. What would you think, feel, and do if you were no longer consumed by anger and resentment? Take time with this before moving on to the next exercise.

The next guided exercise is designed to help you cultivate forgiveness toward yourself and others, allowing you to move forward with a lighter heart and a renewed sense of peace. Before starting, find a candle and a quiet, comfortable space to set it up. This candle will represent someone or an event that caused you pain.

At first, you may find this exercise difficult, especially steps 3 and 4. Be gentle with yourself if it feels overwhelming. Your mind may offer reasons why forgiveness and this exercise is unnecessary. Acknowledge these doubts and be willing to hold them for the sake of living your desired life.

It takes practice and patience to cultivate forgiveness. If you've experienced trauma and struggle with painful memories, consider doing this exercise every other day for several weeks. You can follow along using the audio available at http://www.newharbinger.com/54476. You can also record the text at a slow pace in your own voice and listen to it. Experiment with both options to determine what works best for you.

EXERCISE: The Candle of Forgiveness

Go ahead and light the candle and then get in a comfortable position in your chair. Sit upright with your hands resting in your lap. Your legs can either be uncrossed or crossed, whatever is more comfortable. Allow your eyes to focus on the candle flame and simply watch it.

As you watch the flicker of the candle flame, bring your attention to the gentle rising and falling of your breath in your chest and belly. Like ocean waves coming in and going out, your breath is always there. Notice the rhythm of the breath in your body with each passing inhale… and exhale. Notice the changing patterns of sensations in your belly as you breathe in and as you breathe out. Take a few minutes to center yourself as you breathe in and out.

Step 1: Become Aware of the Wrong and Hurt Beneath the Painful Memory

Now allow your awareness to shift to a painful memory or traumatic event. See if you can allow yourself to visualize the scene fully as if you were watching a movie in slow motion. What happened? Who else was there? Watch the flame as you acknowledge the painful situation unfolding in your mind's eye. Focus on your breathing as you watch the situation unfold. See if you can slow the painful situation down, slower and slower with each passing breath.

As you do, bring your attention to any sensations of discomfort that show up. As best you can, bring an attitude of generous allowing and gentle acceptance to your experience right now. See if you can make room for the pain and hurt you had then and that you may be reliving now. Soften to it…as you breathe in…and out…in…and out.

As best as you can, open up to any hurt, pain, sadness, regret, loss, and resentment. Allow yourself to become aware of your hurt and painful emotions, and simply acknowledge the hurt you experienced and the hurt you may have caused. There's no need to resist or fight or blame. Simply acknowledge and become aware of your experience.

Step 2: Separate Hurtful Actions from Your Hurt and Its Source

Visualize the person or event that inflicted the hurt. As you begin to do so, allow the person or event to drift over and become the candle. If it was you, then see yourself as the candle. Focus on the candle and continue to visualize the person or situation that hurt you or caused the hurt. Now remember and visualize what happened. As you focus on the candle, notice what your mind machine is doing with the images and sensations that show up.

You might see your mind making a judgment...blaming...having feelings of sadness...bitterness...resentment. As these and other thoughts and sensations come into your awareness, simply label them as you did in previous exercises—*There is judgment...blame...tension...resentment*—and allow them to be. Bring a gentle and kind awareness to your pain and hurt as you breathe in...and out...in...and out...slowly and deeply.

Next, create some space between the actions that made you feel hurt and angry and the person or situation that created them. If it helps, you can visualize the action that hurt you as the flame, and the person or situation causing the hurt as the candle. If you were the source of the hurt, then let your actions become the flame and you the candle.

Notice that the flame is not the candle. The actions of the person who hurt you are not the same as the person who committed them. As you breathe in and out, give yourself time to connect with this difference. Then, bring each hurtful action into the flame one by one and notice it, label it, and then see the difference between the hurtful action and the person. Visualize what was done, not who did it.

After you spend some time noticing each action, allow it to disappear up into the smoke, leaving the candle flame. Keep watching any tension, discomfort, anger, hurt, or whatever else your body may be doing. Make room for what you experience as you return your attention to your body and your breathing. Don't try to change or fix anything.

Step 3: Bring Compassionate Witness to Your Hurt

Next, bring your attention back to the human being in the candle—the perpetrator of wrongs against you, or those that you may have committed yourself. Notice how they're also a human being and vulnerable to harm just like you.

See if you can allow yourself to take that person's perspective as a compassionate witness and see what life might be like through their eyes. Connect with that person's hardships, losses, missed opportunities, poor choices, faults and failings, hurts and sadness, and hopes and dreams. Imagine their childhood. Consider what kind of parents or family they must have had. Go further to imagine how their life experiences shaped their view of themself and others, and the world. Consider how their history must have influenced their decisions and actions.

Without condoning their actions, see if you can connect with that person's humanity and imperfections as you connect with your own humanity and imperfections, hardships, loss, pain, and suffering.

As a compassionate witness to this other human being, see if you can connect more deeply with that person, even if that person is you, as another human being. Notice the offender's thoughts and feelings, knowing that you've also experienced similar types of thoughts and feelings. What might it be like to have lived the life of the person who offended you? As best you can, bring an attitude of generous allowing and gentle acceptance to your experience now.

Step 4: Extend Forgiveness, Let Go, and Move On

Now imagine what your life would be like if you released all the negative energy linked with your past—your grievances, grudges, bitterness, and anger. Consider what your life would be like if you were no longer dwelling on past wrongs or if you weren't trying to shut out these painful memories. Connect with the reasons behind your desire to be free from the painful memory, the anger, or the desire for revenge.

Allow yourself to visualize a new future, abundant with opportunities and experiences you've missed by being unwilling to forgive. Connect with this further without forgetting the past, and without carrying the weight of bitterness and anger toward those who hurt you.

Now is the time to take a courageous step forward by letting go of the memory, pain, anger, and resentment. With each exhale, let go of resentment and bitterness, and on each inhale, welcome peace and forgiveness. Feel the relief as you release the burden you've carried for so long. Breathe slowly and deeply, while embracing this new sense of freedom and peace.

When you're ready, reflect on times when you've needed forgiveness from others in the past. Imagine extending that forgiveness to the person who hurt or offended you. What would you say to them? As you consider this, notice any discomfort and observe what your mind is doing.

If thoughts like *They don't deserve forgiveness* or *I don't deserve that* arise, acknowledge them and gently let them go. Then, bring your attention to your breathing as you remind yourself that kind and gentle acts of forgiveness are for your benefit, not others.

Visualize the burden being lifted as you choose to extend forgiveness. Connect with the healing and empowerment that accompanies this choice. Notice the softening of emotions where there was once hardness, hurt, and pain.

Embrace this moment of peace as you visualize the person who offended you, including yourself if necessary. Extend your hands gently and say, "In forgiving you, I forgive myself. By releasing my pain and anger toward you, I will find peace and freedom within myself. I welcome peace and compassion into my life and toward my pain. I choose to let go of this burden I've carried for so long." Repeat these phrases slowly as you offer forgiveness.

Observe and label any thoughts and feelings that arise as you extend forgiveness. Notice the emotional relief as the burden of resentment and bitterness melts away. Feel the peace and inner strength that emerge as you offer compassion and forgiveness in this moment.

Then, when you're ready, bring your awareness back into the room, to your body, and to the flicker of the candle flame. Finish this exercise by blowing out the candle as a symbolic gesture of your commitment to release the past and of your readiness to move on with your life.

LIFE-ENHANCEMENT EXERCISES

We all have something in our past that can haunt us and keep us stuck. Be mindful that you are learning new skills that will help you break free from the bondage of your past so that you can create a new future. This week, we suggest that you spend time with the exercises in this chapter. Do them at your own pace. They need not be done all at once. And be mindful that you're doing this work in the service of living the kind of life you wish to have from this point forward. Remember that the pages of your life book from here on out haven't been written. They can be a repeat of the past or something truly new. You get to decide what goes in there.

THE TAKE-HOME MESSAGE

Your mind is set up to recall events over and over, particularly the nasty ones. That's what modern psychology teaches us. But keeping your eyes fixed on the past is no way to live. You don't need to live your life as a victim of your past—as living proof of all the terrible wrongs that were committed against you. This just hurts you again and again.

As you engage with the exercises in this chapter, remember that you're acquiring tools to break free from the chains of your past. You're also learning that you are more than your past. You control how you will carry your memories forward.

Take your time with these exercises, doing them at your own pace. You don't need to complete them all at once. Keep in mind that you're doing this work to make peace with your past, so you have freedom to create the life you desire moving forward. Your life book is still being written, and you have the power to determine its contents.

Making Peace with My Past So I Can Move On

Reflections:

- My past is part of who I am, but it doesn't define me. I was there before the trauma and dark moments, and I am here now—I am!

- I acknowledge the pain and trauma I've experienced, but I refuse to let it control my present or future. I cannot change what happened, but I have the power to learn from past, make peace with it, and move forward with purpose.

Inquiries:

- Am I willing to make peace with my past? If not, then what's getting in my way?

- Am I allowing myself to be defined by past hurts, or am I ready to break free from that narrative? Am I living my life as a victim, as living proof of past wrongs? Is this serving me well?

- Am I willing to envision a future where I take the lessons of my past without being burdened by them?

- Can I take the bold step to let go and bring compassion, kindness, and forgiveness to my hurt and pain? Am I willing to make room for something new?

CHAPTER 17

Moving Toward a Valued Life

The journey of a thousand miles must begin with a single step.

—Lao Tzu

In the journey of your life, every step matters. Each step will either move you toward or away from what you care about. To navigate life wisely, you must align your actions with your values, those guiding principles that illuminate your path amidst life's challenges. Over time, with these steps you'll create the conditions for genuine happiness and what you end up calling your life.

Values point you in a direction toward what's important. This is crucial when you feel pulled and pushed around in a sea of worry, anxiety, panic, and doom and gloom. The next step is to take control of your actions and start moving in vital directions by focusing on specific goals.

Goals serve as waypoints, marking your progress toward fulfilling your values. Breaking down your values into actionable steps will empower you to live a meaningful life, one step at a time. By committing to these steps, you'll take control of your destiny and craft the life you desire.

Are you ready and willing to take these steps?

SETTING AND ACHIEVING GOALS

Return to the Life Compass you completed in chapter 6. It's time to prioritize which values and intentions you want to nurture in your life right now. Choose a life domain and a value that you've found challenging to act on, possibly due to anxiety-related obstacles. This would be a good place to start. If you sense that you're not yet ready to confront barriers in this important life area, then select a different area and set of values that you're willing to work with.

Once you decide on the value that you want to work with now, write it down at the top of the Value and Goals Worksheet at the end of this chapter. You can also download the worksheet at http://www.newharbinger.com/54476. You'll want to print extra copies of this worksheet for other valued intentions that you'll work on later.

Be SMART with Your Goals

George Doran (1981) developed a very effective five-step behavioral program to help people achieve goals. He called them SMART goals. Though Doran developed the program for people in business, it has been used widely and successfully in ACT (Harris 2008). It can help you do more of what matters to you. Let's go over these steps one by one:

1. **S**pecific—Identify concrete goals on your journey.

2. **M**eaningful—Choose goals that align with your values and aspirations.

3. **A**ctive—Select goals that you can do and that enhance your life satisfaction and well-being.

4. **R**ealistic—Set goals that are attainable given your life circumstances.

5. **T**ime-framed—Establish a timeline for each goal, including when and where you will take a step, and remember to celebrate your progress along the way!

The last important piece here involves practice. Once you set a SMART goal, practice taking the steps to live out your values in situations that have been difficult for you. Repetition builds confidence, as unfamiliar steps that seem scary will become more routine and ordinary over time. Below, we'll walk you through how to set goals and accomplish them.

Identify Concrete and Achievable Goals

As you start thinking about goals, consider your short-term and long-term objectives, as each contributes to progress on your valued path. Short-term goals provide immediate milestones, while long-term goals offer a broader vision to strive for. Let's consider an example.

Suppose you value your health and one of your valued intentions is to increase your fitness level. So, you commit to walking each day. Your long-term goal might be to walk to a telephone pole one mile from where you live. Between your house and that pole are several other poles, all spaced about the same distance apart.

An initial short-term goal might be getting to the first pole. The next day you commit to getting to both the first and the second pole, and so on. If you keep at it, you'll eventually reach your one-mile marker—your long-term goal. This is how short- and long-term goals work—they get and keep you moving on a valued path.

To get and stay moving, it's important that you avoid ending up on a dead-end street. Setting goals is all about workability. If you don't make your goals workable in the context of your life, it's unlikely you're going to get very far. Choose achievable actions that reflect your values and realistically fit your life circumstances. This will make it more likely that you'll follow through and live your values every day.

In the space below, write down some goals related to the first valued intention you have chosen to work on from your Life Compass. Be sure your goals are concrete and specific.

To help you get concrete, ask yourself this: *What would other people see me doing? How would they know I have done something new?* Focus on one or a few things you can do with your mouth, hands, and feet. And be sure you will be able to tick them off your to-do list once you complete them:

We suggest that you start with one or two goals. One should be a short-term SMART goal—something you can start working on this week. Then ask the following SMART goal questions for each goal to make sure it's achievable:

- Is the goal **specific** (concrete, practical)?

- Is it **meaningful** (reflects what truly matters to me)?

- Is it **active** (something I can do and have control over)?

- Is it **realistic** (does it work with my current life situation)?

- Is it **time-framed** (can I put in on my calendar and do it)?

Above all, be sure that your goal aligns with your valued intention: does it express what matters to you? If it does, then you've crafted a good SMART goal. If not, then go back and rework your SMART goal. Think small. What tiny step could you take that would reflect your values and move you toward the life you desire?

If necessary, revise and clarify the goal until you can answer yes to each SMART goal question above.

Once your SMART goal is clear, write it down on the Value and Goals Worksheet.

Identify Steps and Arrange Them in Logical Order

Now that you've established your goals, it's time to outline the incremental steps needed to reach them. Begin with your short-term goal and break it down into smaller intermediate steps. Identify each action required to achieve your goal and write these actions here or on a separate piece of paper:

Now, consider the logical sequence for these steps. Determine what needs to occur first before you can move ahead with the others. If no particular order is required, begin with the easiest step. Then, transfer the steps into the Value and Goals Worksheet in the sequence you will complete them. Repeat this process for other goals you've identified.

Let's look at an example. Suppose your goal is to spend quality time with your spouse or partner. To get there, you may identify several intermediate steps, including activities you both enjoy, like going to a movie, dining out, making time to catch up, or taking a bike ride together. You may then commit to doing at least one quality-time activity with your partner each week. Notice that there's no logical order to the steps in this example. What's important is that you do these things regardless of what your mind is thinking or how you feel.

Make a Commitment and Take the Step

Now, it's time to commit. Are you ready to embrace the values you explored in chapters 5 and 6 and the life changes they entail? If so, choose a specific day and time to begin step 1 on your Value and Goals Worksheet. Share this commitment with someone else. Then, regardless of how you feel at the time, take action. Remember, change requires action. Without it, nothing will improve. You'll continue to get what you've always gotten.

Record the date on the worksheet when you accomplish each step. Put a gold star on a calendar if you want to. Make sure to celebrate your progress, no matter how small the step. Review your Value and Goals Worksheet on a regular basis. It will give you valuable feedback on your progress and will help you stay motivated as you check off your goals.

KNOWING YOUR BARRIERS

All along you've been gaining clarity about internal barriers that get in the way of living your life, and you've been working to change your relationship with them. But external barriers may also pose challenges, such as financial constraints, time limitations, lack of skills or information, or conflicts over what other people want, need, or expect.

The good news is that it doesn't really matter if the barriers are inside or outside of you. The key is to develop a plan to address and move forward with them. You'll find examples of how two of our former clients, Jill and Eric, completed the Value and Goals Worksheet, at http://www.newharbinger.com/54476.

The next exercise will help you anticipate barriers and challenges that might get in the way of acting on your value-guided SMART goals. This will allow you to create a plan, using all the skills you've been practicing so far, to approach these barriers, so you can keep moving forward.

So, let's take a moment to settle and get clear about the barriers you might face as you act on your value-guided goal. You can follow along using the audio at http://www.newharbinger.com/54476.

EXERCISE: Anticipating Barriers

Just take a moment to close your eyes and bring to mind one of your valued intentions—the things you care about in your heart and want to be about. Sink into the sweetness of that—the sense of lining up with your core. If that's hard to do, imagine for a moment that nothing gets in your way and that you're free to do what you really, truly care about. See yourself being about something that matters in your heart.

Now, see yourself living out those intentions as if watching yourself on a giant movie screen. Focus on the very first step or two just as you decide to act. Notice where you are. Notice what you're saying. Notice what you're doing with your hands and feet. And, if other people are involved, watch how they might be responding to you. And now, take an inventory of what's showing up inside of you.

Observe what your mind is telling you. Is there judgment of you or the situation or other people? Do you notice blocking thoughts, like *I can't do this…it's too much*? Or, discouraging thoughts, like *Nothing matters…so don't bother*. Or, maybe your mind is conjuring up images of catastrophe, old wounds, doom and gloom, or maybe it's telling you something else like *I don't have enough time*. Just notice what's there and take stock.

Now move on to what's going on in your body. What are you feeling? And, if observing what you're feeling is still difficult for you, see if you can notice any sense of hardening, closing down, or pulling back. As you observe, notice what's showing up just as it is, like *I'm noticing hardening*, *tensing*, or *shutting down*.

Also, see if you can detect any physical sensations in your body such as tension, energy, or your heart pounding, or maybe you're holding your breath or breathing really fast. Just take stock of that too and observe it.

Now look and see if your mind is commanding you to do something. Is it telling you to cut and run, turn away, lash out, or give up? Just notice these urges and impulses and ride the wave.

And, if we've left anything out, just notice what that may be in your experience. It could be thoughts, emotions, sensations, or urges to act or react. Look to the barriers you've been working on to guide you here. Some may arise within you, others may be external to you.

As you wrap up this exercise, come back to where you are right now, and allow yourself one or two deep breaths in and out. And then, slowly open your eyes.

Use what you learned from the imagery exercise you just did, or look to your past experiences, to anticipate barriers that may show up as you step in directions that matter. Write them down on the Value and Goals Worksheet. Then, consider how you can leverage the skills you've acquired from this book to approach those barriers. Importantly, write down the skills you plan to use to keep yourself moving forward when barriers show up, as they undoubtedly will.

Maybe it's dropping the rope, mindfulness, grounding, taking the observer perspective, writing thoughts on cards, saying to yourself *I'm having the thought that…*, or any of the other skills. Remember, look to the exercises, metaphors, and images that you've found helpful so far.

We encourage you to take your time with this part. You need to have a plan to approach your internal barriers in a new way. Without a plan, you risk falling back into old patterns that didn't work before and that probably won't work in the future. As we've talked about in previous chapters, repeating old and unhelpful behaviors will give you old and unhelpful outcomes.

EMBRACING YOUR VALUES: REWARDS AND CHALLENGES

The next two exercises will help you get in touch with the immediate challenges and rewards that living your values can offer you. Again, for the first few times, we recommend listening to the audio at http://www.newharbinger.com/54476.

EXERCISE: The Rewards of Living Your Values

Go ahead and close your eyes and take a few slow breaths as you center yourself. Now bring to mind the valued intention you worked with in the previous exercise about anticipating barriers. Once you have that valued intention in mind, see yourself acting on that value just as you wish *and* with nothing standing in your way. You're free of barriers and successful in doing what you set out to do.

Notice what you're doing and sink into the sweetness of this moment, this experience, just as you might linger with a beautiful sunset. What does success feel like on the inside? Notice any thoughts, emotions, and physical sensations. See if you can touch a sense of satisfaction, a sense that you're doing something good for yourself and your life too.

Stay with this image, and when you're ready, shift your attention to the world around you— the people, the events, and the environment that surround you in this scenario. What's different? Become aware of how people in the situation are reacting to you and to what you've accomplished. How does it feel to be freed from an old barrier? How does it feel to freely do something you've been afraid to do? Notice how the situation changes for the better because of what you did in the service of your values.

Stay with this exercise, this experience, for as long as you wish. And, when you're ready to wrap up, open your eyes, and then grab a piece of paper and jot down any positive outcomes you discovered during this exercise. Use them as a reminder of the possibilities ahead as you begin your journey with the Value and Goals Worksheet.

In the next exercise, we'll ask you to shift your awareness to what's possible as you act on your values in situations where one of your WAF barriers shows up. This exercise will help you see how you can uphold your values even when it is difficult to do so.

EXERCISE: **Creating a Success Story**

Get comfortable and take a few slow, deep breaths. Allow your eyes to close gently. And, when you're ready, bring to mind one of your values that's been difficult for you to act on because of your anxiety barriers—you can use the same value as before or a different one. When you have it in mind, imagine that you're taking just one step to act on that value. See the very first thing you'd say or do as if you were watching yourself on a movie screen. See your actions and hear your words.

As you do, see and hear how others respond to you as you watch the scene unfold. What are they saying? What are they doing?

And then kindly observe any barriers that show up inside you. See if you can notice emotions that seem to block you from taking another step to support your values. Notice any thoughts that are trying to thwart you on this path. Do the same with any physical sensations in your body. Continue to watch and observe your thoughts, feelings, and physical sensations without resistance.

Open up to them, allow them to be, however scary or unpleasant they might seem. Notice the wave of emotion and remind yourself that sooner or later it will crest and then recede. So, stay with yourself and ride it out. As you do, be kind with your mind and body and experience. Soften to the barriers with each breath, creating more space for you to be right where you are.

Now come back to the scene and see yourself completing what you set out to do. Sink into the satisfaction of doing what you care about, and every good thing that happens for you, for others, and for your world. Notice any sense of sweetness in that. Acknowledge that you did something good for yourself and your life even though it was difficult to do.

Both exercises aim to shift your focus to what's achievable and possible in your life. Every barrier essentially says, "You can't do this" or "You can't have this," but buying into these thoughts prevents you from pursuing what truly matters. We saw this dynamic play out with one of our sons, Aidan, during Little League.

At the time, Aidan was in a batting slump, and he was quite hard on himself because of it. During batting practice, he'd quickly get frustrated and say, "I can't hit this stupid ball!" This mindset extended to his game performance, where he stopped swinging at pitches. It got to the point where going to the field for practice became a chore.

In a way, Aidan faced an impossible situation. While trying to bat, he listened to his mind's insistence that he "can't hit." How's he going to hit a baseball when he's focused on not hitting?

So, after explaining the situation to Aidan's coach, we found a solution: Aidan was encouraged to imagine himself hitting the ball and experiencing the joy and satisfaction that might follow. This is what helped him break out of his batting slump! You can do that too.

But you need to have a clear image of what it is you want to do, where you want to go, and the possible rewards of acting in ways that matter to you. That's why SMART goals are so important. They are the steps along the path into the life you wish to create. Just be sure you give yourself time to practice as much as you need.

LIFE-ENHANCEMENT EXERCISES

- Practice valued living by following the steps outlined in this chapter. Use the Value and Goals Worksheet to plan activities and to prepare for the difficulties and barriers that may come up along the way. Start with one value and a set of related goals. Later, you can work on other values and goals in a similar fashion.

- Practice the exercises that will help you visualize and make contact with the rewards of living out your values, even when WAF barriers show up.

- Also continue to practice any of the earlier exercises in this book as often as possible, including practicing kindness toward yourself, particularly when anxiety shows up during the day. Every exercise in this book will help you move in directions that matter to you.

THE TAKE-HOME MESSAGE

To change your life, you'll need to commit to changing what you do, pure and simple. You can get back on the road to a valued life by focusing on your values, setting goals, and then taking action, no matter how you feel or what you're thinking. Acceptance, compassion, and kindness will be your friends when you deal with barriers that will undoubtedly come up.

Putting My Values into Action

Reflections:

- Each day offers an opportunity to align my actions with my values, even amidst challenges. I can live my values by setting concrete and achievable SMART goals.

- Making small, consistent commitments to living my values—even in difficult situations—is the essence of progress.

Inquiries:

- How can I translate my values into daily actions?

- What steps can I take to break down my goals into manageable tasks that I can tackle one at a time?

Value and Goals Worksheet

My valued intention:			
SMART goal I want to achieve:			
Steps toward achieving my goal	Barriers	Strategies	Date(s) achieved
1.			
2.			
3.			
4.			
5.			

CHAPTER 18

The Journey Ahead

Where you end up isn't the most important thing. It's the road you take to get there. The road you take is what you'll look back on and call your life.

—Tim Wiley

Life is not a destination. It's a journey—and one that you'll look back on someday and call your life. This way of looking at things demands a shift in focus.

When you started this book, you may have been looking to tackle your anxieties and fears first so that you could then be happy and thrive once you started feeling better. We hope that you've learned by now that this is not the solution but a recipe for more suffering.

This is why we've encouraged you to put your attention on learning the skills for changing your relationship with your mind and body first, with the purpose of making the most out of the life you have and in ways that you care about.

This shift in focus is exactly how you create genuine happiness. And yes, you deserve to be genuinely happy. You deserve to be free of needless suffering. You can cultivate genuine happiness by practicing being gentle, kind, mindful, and defused, and by being more willing, open, and allowing with your mind, body, and everything your history throws at you. These are the skills that will create genuine happiness and peace. We hope that by now you're starting to connect with this basic truth—a truth that's now supported by quite a bit of research, as we discussed in the prologue.

So here, we'd like to congratulate you for all the work you've done and will continue to do. You've come a long way! But there's still more to do—fortunately, your journey isn't over yet. Our wish is that you'll keep yourself moving forward in ways that matter to you, long after you put down this book.

HOW TO KEEP ON MOVING

As you embark on your journey of putting your values into action, there will be new obstacles, doubts, and setbacks. The old WAF obstacles and your old responses to them will show up too. At times, you won't put your commitments into actions. Sometimes you'll slip into old WAF habits. Occasionally, it will take longer to reach a goal than you'd hoped. All of this and more is just fine. Living your life is not a horse race. We all move at our own pace.

The most important thing is to keep yourself moving forward in meaningful ways. You can draw upon the strategies and skills you've learned in previous chapters for how to respond when *difficulty* threatens to get in the way of *vitality*.

Practice Your Skills

The first and most important recommendation we have for you is simple: keep practicing the skills you've learned in this book. Just as with any skill, you need to use these skills regularly or you'll risk losing them. Many people revert to old, familiar, and unhelpful habits because they stop applying the skills they've learned in programs like this one.

So, make a commitment to practice an exercise or two daily in a quiet place, and use your skills in your daily life. Download the audio exercises from the website for this book and make them part of your daily routine. Your practice doesn't have to be long or drawn out—even five to twenty minutes a day can be helpful. The key is to keep the skills alive by using them. The more you use them, the more they'll become a habit that will alter the trajectory of your life for the better.

Stick with the exercises and metaphors that have been particularly helpful in getting you unstuck and moving forward. Revisit them and focus on them. Also, try experimenting with one or two exercises that you haven't tried yet, and see how they impact your life.

As you work to apply your new skills in your daily life, you may find it helpful to reflect on any remaining WAF sticky spots—thoughts, images, memories, bodily sensations, urges, and situations that keep you stuck—and then focus your mindful acceptance and observer self-practice on them. If you ever feel discouraged, revisit your valued-life epitaph—you could even rework or expand it!

Recommit After Breaking a Commitment

There will be times when you commit to value-guided action and, for whatever reason, fail to follow through. Often, this stems from old and new barriers showing up. We're pretty sure that the passengers on your Life Bus will be shouting things like "You'll never make it!" or "You're going to make a fool of yourself!" or "See, you still felt panicky after all this work you did!"

You know that following through with a commitment can be challenging when faced with WAFs. But here, it's crucial to remember that you can always recommit to taking actions that align with your values and your life.

Expect barriers, uncertainty, and doubt, as your mind may not always offer helpful advice. In fact, your mind will likely conjure up all sorts of doubts, fears, and reasons to discourage you from taking action. During these times, come back to this key question: *Am I willing to commit fully to this activity in the service of my values?*

This is a choice only you can make, and we hope you will, again and again. Knowing that you're bound to experience discomfort and doubt, are you still willing to commit 100 percent to this or that activity and follow through? Remember, commitment isn't something you can try or do halfway. You either make the commitment or you don't.

We're not asking you to commit to success or any other particular outcome like "being in a steady relationship by a certain date" or "feeling better and less anxious." Many outcomes are beyond your control. They lie somewhere in the future and can only be known *after* you've taken a step. We're only asking whether you're willing to commit to doing something that will work for you *and* while taking all passengers with you on your Life Bus. Will you do that and mean it?

Commitment means choosing to act in the present moment. It doesn't mean you'll never fall short; we all do. When that happens, learn from it, pick yourself up, and recommit to action.

GETTING BACK ON TRACK IS WHAT COUNTS!

Remember, a valued life is built on SMART goals, one step at a time, one moment after the next. Each day offers another opportunity to act on your SMART goals. Your choices and actions ultimately determine what happens with barriers and setbacks on your road to valued living. At times, all of us will fail to live consistently with our values. What happens next is critical.

When you fall short, make a choice to recommit to stay on the path of your values. Let go of buying into the failure judgment and being strangled by it—just put it on a card and take it along. And then make a renewed commitment to take actions that move you in life directions you care about.

When you let a WAF barrier stop you from time to time, don't slide into thinking that this means that WAFs will take over your life again. That won't happen unless *you* allow it to happen. It's your choice to either give up or recommit to small actions that make your life meaningful—and then put those actions into practice. So long as you do that and keep moving, you'll be truly living a life that expresses your values.

This entire book has been about helping you make life-affirming choices—every day and every moment of your life. If you've worked the exercises so far, then you're not the same person you were when you first cracked open this book.

Move with Barriers and Setbacks

Remember that you don't need to overcome worry, anxiety, or fears before moving forward on the road to living your values. You don't need to get rid of them. And, you don't have to change them either.

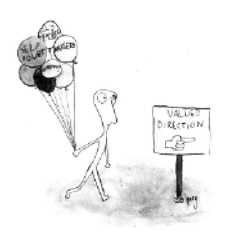

The key is to acknowledge the barriers and move *with* them—take them along with you like you see in the image to your left. Let your values show you the way. Make room for all the unwanted stuff. Don't let it stop you from doing what's best for you. Keep on nurturing your willingness to have what you have, and stop running from yourself.

Focus on changing your relationship with your mind, body, spirit, and life right now, in this moment and then the next. You and you alone are the driver of your Life Bus. To have the life you want, you need to keep yourself in the driver's seat and carry all the passengers with you, both pleasant and unpleasant.

Unpleasant passengers will be the most challenging, but there are other passengers who need your attention because they'll remind you of what you care about and want in your life.

When in doubt, do the opposite of what WAFs tell you to do. Don't listen to Anxiety News Radio; tune in to Just So Radio by watching what's going on from your kind and gentle observer perspective. Cherish the moment as it is! It too will pass.

And don't forget to watch what's going on inside you with some kindness and compassion. Nurturing friendliness and willingness will make it easier to move with your WAFs. They're not your enemy but more like a wounded child who needs some care and kindness. Take care of that child. Embrace it. Take it with you on your journey.

Don't Let the Mind Machine Trap You

The mind machine won't stop its chatter just because you've made a commitment to act and to take your WAFs with you when they show up. When you fall short of being accepting and following through with your commitments, your judgmental mind may scorn you: *Stop all this acceptance and commitment BS. You just can't do it. The only thing you should accept is that you're a failure at acceptance and commitment!*

When your mind throws old, unhelpful, sticky stuff at you, don't get tangled up in the chatter. This is just another example of your mind doing what minds do all the time: creating thoughts and evaluating. It's just more "blah, blah, blah."

Ask yourself if the "blah, blah, blah" is really helpful to you. Do you need to listen and trust all those thoughts your mind baits you with? Must you argue with "blah, blah, blah"? Or can you make room for these thoughts and let them be? This will free you up to move on with your life, no matter how strong the feelings, no matter how loud the thoughts. These are the times when you need to watch your mind machine in action, as you've learned to do.

Here, the practice is always the same: willingly acknowledge and observe your mind doing its thing, without struggling or buying into everything it comes up with. This is how to drop the old unhelpful story lines.

With time, you'll get better at noticing when you're hooked and when your mind is helpful. This important skill will empower you to move forward with whatever your mind offers you.

Watch for Idleness and Fill It with Active Vitality

When you sit on your hands doing nothing, you create a vast void in your mind. Your mind, in turn, will do what it can to fill this empty space, often with judgments, criticisms, dire predictions, and old barriers. You've probably noticed this yourself, especially if you've struggled with anticipatory anxiety. These times can be high-risk situations for getting hooked. Idleness is a great setup for Anxiety News Radio.

You have two ways to go from here. One is to get mired in unhelpful and self-limiting thoughts and do nothing. The other is to welcome what shows up as it is and ask yourself, *What can I do right now that aligns with my values?* or *What do I want to be about as a person right now?* We think this latter option is better for you.

Take action, no matter how small, to clear out the mental clutter and move forward on your life journey. That's how to make your life grow.

Practice Flexibility

Each time you step out of your comfort zone, you enhance your flexibility. You become more open, adaptable, and ready to embrace new experiences. This growth enriches your life and allows you to learn and grow into the person you wish to become.

There are several ways to practice flexibility. Here are a few suggestions:

- **Freshen up your mindfulness and meditation practice.** You can do this by switching between the different types of exercises in this book and on the companion website (http://www.newharbinger.com/54476). You can also practice the exercises in different places or settings. In addition, you can find new exercises in print or online, including various apps. Or you can create new exercises yourself.

- **When you're stuck in a rut, step out of that rut and do something new.** One of our clients noticed that every time he'd go out to dinner, he'd order the same thing—steak. It didn't matter where he went. He finally decided to consider the whole menu and choose something different. He now enjoys crab. Life is like a menu too. It gives you many offerings. Look for them, step out of your ruts, and follow your bliss.

- **Continue reading and learning.** Check out the list of further readings and helpful internet resources provided at http://www.newharbinger.com/54476 to refresh and expand your knowledge about mindfulness, meditation, and the ACT approach to anxiety and other related concerns. We have also created a smaller and much shorter pocket-size book entitled *Anxiety Happens* (Forsyth and Eifert 2018) and *The Anxiety Happens Guided Journal* (Forsyth and Eifert 2023). Both books offer more condensed coverage of the concepts and exercises contained in this more detailed workbook. You might find them useful as a refresher from time to time.

- **Feed your mind and life with uplifting news and experiences.** If you're the type of person who's glued to the news, the internet, social media, or other sources of stimulation, it might be a good idea to do a media detox. Give yourself a break—quiet time away from the negative noise of the world around you. Turn off the TV, your phone, and the radio, and do something you value. Stillness creates opportunities for peace and gives you space to think and move. You can fill that stillness with something other than negative news and social media hype. Fill it with valued action, uplifting information, beautiful nature, music, a hobby. The most effective way to dispel darkness is to bring in the light.

- **Nurture a spirit of playfulness with your mind, body, and life.** Kids are masters at the art of play, and we seem to lose that as we grow up. But study after study shows that adults who practice being more playful with themselves and others, and make time for fun and play, are generally happier and healthier, and live longer too. Perhaps you've left play on the back burner for a very long time. That's fine. There are lots of ways you can bring it back into your life. Think about the things you like to do that are fun, and see if you can build a spirit of play into your life. You can also bring the spirit of playfulness to your mind and emotional life. You don't need to take your thoughts, feelings, and physical sensations so seriously. Of course, see a doctor if you're seriously ill or injured. But that's not what we're dealing with here when it comes to your WAFs. Embody a spirit of lightheartedness with yourself and others, and you may be pleasantly surprised at what it offers you.

Build Your Willingness Muscle

Life is about asking whether you're *willing* to be open to any difficulties inside your skin, and in the world around you, in the service of living a life that matters to you. You already have a sense of what willingness is like. It's not the absence of fear but the decision that something else is more important than the fear. This, by the way, is how we've come to think about courage too.

You decide to step, and step again, with your arms wide open. You'll never be certain about what you may find, but you can rest in the sweetness of knowing that you stepped in ways that uphold and honor your values.

You've already gained a new perspective and powerful skills to navigate life's challenges while staying true to your values. Your past doesn't define you; it's how you handle challenges going forward that shapes your future.

Above all, remember that you control your willingness switch. When old WAFs try to take over your Life Bus, ask yourself, *Am I willing to engage in my life now, whatever that might bring, in the service of doing what matters to me?* If yes, then take a leap and trust that you have everything you need to move forward.

Want Something More Than Comfort and Safety

We've covered this already, but it's worth revisiting. You need to want something more than "not feeling anxious." You need to desire something bigger than relative comfort and safety. Otherwise, you will not act. When faced with choices, you'll choose the path of least resistance, even though it's deadening.

So, when you think about your life and your choices, want something more than what you've always got. Chart a new course. Experiment. But above all, move your values from your head down to your heart and gut. This is what Larry, one of our former clients, did.

When Larry first came to see us, he was terrified of driving on backcountry roads and would avoid them at all costs. But he also said that he valued his marriage and would do anything for his partner. One day, Larry's partner called him, very upset. She told him that while out driving, she had swerved to miss hitting a deer, and her car had ended up in a ditch at the end of a rural country road some distance from where they lived. She needed his help.

Larry's old fear screamed, "No, you can't go…you might get stuck out there!" But his values screamed even louder. He later told us that he got in his car and raced over to help her, and he was glad he did. He added that it was difficult and nothing would have kept him from coming to the aid of his partner—even his fear of driving backcountry roads.

This is what we mean by wanting something more than comfort and safety. When you look at your life and your values, make sure you find that heartfelt something.

Are You Moving Forward or Backward in Your Life?

When facing barriers and you're unsure what to do, pause and ask yourself, *Is my response moving me closer to or further away from where I want to go in life?* Below are some variations of this crucial question that your life is asking:

- If that thought, emotion, bodily state, or memory could give advice, would it point me forward in my life or keep me stuck?

- What advice would my core value of _____ give me right now?

- What would I advise my child or someone else to do in this situation?

- If others could see what I'm doing now, would they see me doing things that align with my values?

- What do I have control over right now?

- When I listen to my WAFs, where do I end up?

- What does my experience tell me about this solution? And what do I trust more—my mind and feelings or my lived experience?

Asking these questions when faced with adversity and doubt is more helpful than listening to unwise WAF thoughts or impulses. The answers will remind you that past solutions haven't worked, giving you the chance to decide to do something differently.

EMOTIONAL DISCOMFORT IS YOUR TEACHER

WAFs and other sources of emotional pain and hurt are often viewed as enemies when, in fact, they're teachers. Think about that for a moment.

Without experiencing disappointment, you'd never learn to hold your expectations about the future more lightly. Without the ability to experience hurt, you'd never learn kindness and compassion. Without frustration and delay, you'd never learn patience. Without loss and grief, you'd never know what love is. Without exposure to new information, you'd never learn anything new.

In a similar way, fear teaches courage and self-compassion. The presence of anxiety may be there because you're not living in alignment with your values and need to change course. Even sickness has its purpose, strengthening immunity and helping you appreciate good health.

Moments of adversity provide you with opportunities for growth and change. They teach you important skills. They give you a fresh perspective on life. They might even help you build resilience. You need them.

When unpleasant feelings arise, they'll often divert attention from what you can control. When that happens, pivot toward your actions and identify what you can control to meet your needs and move forward in meaningful directions. Later, you can develop a specific plan to navigate adversity much like you did when anticipating WAF barriers.

We suggest you apply your compassionate observer skills to each of your painful experiences when you have them. You can choose to open your arms and embrace them when they show up, and bring compassion and forgiveness to them. When you do that, your WAFs lose their power to make you suffer and limit your life. This stance toward your discomfort will also create the conditions for genuine happiness to flourish within you!

A MEANINGFUL LIFE IS BUILT ONE STEP AT A TIME

Sitting still with your WAFs and not getting tangled up with them is one of the toughest parts of practicing courage on a day-to-day basis, and so is letting go of the internal dialogue and struggle. Over time, you'll get more skilled, so long as you keep practicing loving-kindness toward your own slipups, limitations, and all-too-human inability to be perfect.

Begin each day with this commitment: *Today, to the best of my ability, I'm going to act with kindness and courage.* Then follow that with an intention to make your day a value-rich day. In the evening, go back and examine your day with loving-kindness. Don't beat yourself up if your day ends up being filled with some of the same old things you've always done. Look for the new and vital things you did do that day.

Compassion, acceptance, flexibility, and courage are skills and powerful antidotes to suffering. Recognize that you're only human and that you're going to make mistakes and experience setbacks. You're never going to be able to be courageous and accepting all the time; and still, you keep moving in directions you care about, one day at a time.

What matters is taking steps to bring acceptance and compassion for yourself and your worries, anxieties, and fears. These small steps eventually add up, leading to loving-kindness and patience becoming habits in your life. Give yourself time.

Working through this book in the span of several weeks or a few months is not the end of something. It's the beginning of a new chapter in your life. Take your time becoming familiar with all the exercises in this book, so you can more skillfully keep yourself moving in valued directions. And the work isn't over with this book. Your life journey takes a lifetime.

Change is risky, we know. Things might not go as planned, and there's always uncertainty about the future. Yet the biggest risk in life is avoiding risk altogether. If you always play it safe, nothing will change, and you'll remain stuck in a cycle of suffering. You can count on that.

When you risk living your life fully, the payoff is huge—you'll get more of what you want. You'll risk living out your dreams.

THE CHOICE IS YOURS

We'd like to end with what we call the "life question." It's by far the most important question that life is asking you when you're faced with obstacles, problems, and pain.

At those times, stop, take a deep breath or two, and ask yourself this simple question: *Am I willing to do what matters to me in this moment with whatever life offers?*

We all need to face this question squarely and be willing to answer it, one moment after the next, for as long as we're alive.

Saying yes is the only answer that will help you create a life aligned with your values. In fact, when you say yes, you're affirming that anxiety is no longer a barrier. In those moments you're no longer living the life of someone with an anxiety disorder. You are free.

A "no" answer to the life question means only one thing: you're choosing not to live the life you desire. But here's an empowering truth: you can always choose to change your answer. You can take a bold step on a new path and risk doing something new to create a life in line with your deepest longing.

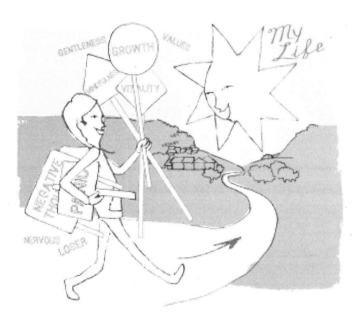

When you started this book, you may have hoped for a magic solution to overcome your anxiety. We've done our best to show you that you don't need a golden shovel to dig yourself out of your anxiety hole. We hope that by now you're seeing this first-hand, moving forward just like you see in the image below from chapter 1. If you need to, go back and review that cartoon series in chapter 1 and reflect on just how far you've come.

The key to creating a meaningful life is not the absence of anxiety but rather your decision to make the most of each moment. You don't have to fight anxiety to have the life you want. Instead, use your skills.

When you wish to avoid something, open up and practice acceptance of experiences over which you have no control. When your mind is unhelpful, notice thoughts as thoughts, stories about you as stories, and let them be. Shift to being an observer of your mind and body. Focus on your values too, for they are your wise and trusty friends. These skills will keep you on the right path.

Make each moment count. Use your time wisely. There's no going back, no do-overs, and no way to save the lost moments of today for tomorrow. In the end, it all adds up to what you'll call your life. Make it about something bigger than your anxiety.

We know you can do it. You have the skills. Continue to nurture them. Allow them to grow. Make your values a reality. This is what matters and what, in the end, leads people to say, "Now there was a life lived well."

Staying the Course for the Long Haul

Reflections:

- Staying committed to living my values means acknowledging and accepting my WAFs and not allowing them to dictate my path. My biggest hurdles are often those that my mind creates. I need to not let them stand in the way of where I wish to go with my life.

- I am at a point now where I can refuse to let WAFs obstruct my journey toward a life aligned with what truly matters to me.

Inquiries:

- Am I at a point where I am ready to draw a line in the sand and say "no more" to anxiety controlling me?

- How can I best keep on moving with my barriers toward a valued life? When I look at what I'm doing right now, is it a move toward or away from my values?

- Am I actively and willingly engaging in activities that resonate with who I want to be?

References

Akbari, M., M. Seydavi, Z. S. Hosseini, J. Krafft, and M. E. Levin. 2022. "Experiential Avoidance in Depression, Anxiety, Obsessive-Compulsive Related, and Post-Traumatic Stress Disorders: A Comprehensive Systematic Review and Meta-Analysis." *Journal of Contextual Behavioral Science* 24: 65–78.

American Psychiatric Association. 2022. *Diagnostic and Statistical Manual of Mental Disorders*, 5th ed., text rev. (DSM-5-TR). Washington, DC: American Psychiatric Association.

Antony, M. M., and R. E. McCabe. 2004. 10 *Simple Solutions to Panic: How to Overcome Panic Attacks, Calm Physical Symptoms, and Reclaim Your Life.* Oakland, CA: New Harbinger Publications.

Arch, J. J., G. H. Eifert, C. Davies, J. C. Plumb Vilardaga, R. D. Rose, and M. G. Craske. 2012. "Randomized Clinical Trial of Cognitive Behavioral Therapy (CBT) Versus Acceptance and Commitment Therapy (ACT) for Mixed Anxiety Disorders." *Journal of Consulting and Clinical Psychology* 80(5): 750–765.

Arikian, S. R., and J. M. Gorman. 2001. "A Review of the Diagnosis, Pharmacologic Treatment, and Economic Aspects of Anxiety Disorders." *Primary Care Companion Journal of Clinical Psychiatry* 3(3): 110–117.

Assagioli, R. 1973. *The Act of Will.* New York: Penguin Books.

Bandelow, B., R. Boerner, S. Kasper, M. Linden, H. U. Wittchen, and H. J. MÖller. 2013. "The Diagnosis and Treatment of Generalized Anxiety Disorder." *Deutsches Ärzteblatt* 1110: 300–310.

Bandelow, B., and S. Michaelis. 2015. "Epidemiology of Anxiety Disorders in the 21st Century." *Dialogues in Clinical Neuroscience* 17(3): 327–335.

Barlow, D. H. 2004. *Anxiety and Its Disorders: The Nature and Treatment of Anxiety and Panic*, 2nd ed. New York: Guilford Press.

Benjet, C., E. Bromet, E. G. Karam, R. C. Kessler, K. A. McLaughlin, A. M. Ruscio, V. Shahly, et al. 2016. "The Epidemiology of Traumatic Event Exposure Worldwide: Results from the World Mental Health Survey Consortium." *Psychological Medicine* 46: 327–343.

Bluett, E. J., K. J. Homan, K. L. Morrison, M. E. Levin, and M. P. Twohig. 2014. "Acceptance and Commitment Therapy for Anxiety and OCD Spectrum Disorders: An Empirical Review." *Journal of Anxiety Disorders* 28(6): 612–624.

Borkovec, T. D., O. Alcaine, and E. Behar. 2004. "Avoidance Theory of Worry and Generalized Anxiety Disorder." In *Generalized Anxiety Disorder: Advances in Research and Practice*, edited by R. G. Heimberg, C. L. Turk, and D. S. Mennin. New York: Guilford Press.

Brach, T. 2004. *Radical Acceptance: Embracing Your Life with the Heart of a Buddha.* New York: Bantam Books.

Caletti, E., C. Massimo, S. Magliocca, C. Moltrasio, P. Brambilla, and G. Delvecchio. 2022. "The Role of the Acceptance and Commitment Therapy in the Treatment of Social Anxiety: An Updated Scoping Review." *Journal of Affective Disorders* 310: 174–182.

Chödrön, P. 2001. *The Places That Scare You: A Guide to Fearlessness in Difficult Times.* Boston: Shambhala Publications.

Chopra, D. 2003. *The Spontaneous Fulfillment of Desire.* New York: Harmony Books.

Conroy, K., J. E. Curtiss, A. L. Barthel, R. Lubin, S. Wieman, E. Bui, N. M. Simon, and S. G. Hofmann. 2020. "Emotion Regulation Flexibility in Generalized Anxiety Disorder." *Journal of Psychopathology and Behavioral Assessment* 42: 93–100.

Coto-Lesmes, R., C. Fernández-Rodríguez, and S. González-Fernández. 2020. "Acceptance and Commitment Therapy in Group Format for Anxiety and Depression. A Systematic Review." *Journal of Affective Disorders* 263: 107–120.

Dahl, J., and T. Lundgren. 2006. *Living Beyond Your Pain: Using Acceptance and Commitment Therapy to Ease Chronic Pain.* Oakland, CA: New Harbinger Publications.

De Castella, K., M. J. Platow, M. Tamir, and J. J. Gross. 2018. "Beliefs About Emotion: Implications for Avoidance-Based Emotion Regulation and Psychological Health." *Cognition and Emotion* 32(4): 773–795.

Doran, G. T. 1981. "There's a S.M.A.R.T. Way to Write Management's Goals and Objectives." *Management Review* 70: 35–36.

Dryman, M. T., and R. G. Heimberg. 2018. "Emotion Regulation in Social Anxiety and Depression: A Systematic Review of Expressive Suppression and Cognitive Reappraisal." *Clinical Psychology Review* 65: 17–42.

Dyer, W. 2012. *Wishes Fulfilled: Mastering the Art of Manifesting.* New York: Hay House.

Eifert, G. H., and M. Heffner. 2003. "The Effects of Acceptance Versus Control Contexts on Avoidance of Panic-Related Symptoms." *Journal of Behavior Therapy and Experimental Psychiatry* 34(3–4): 293–312.

Eifert, G. H., M. McKay, and J. P. Forsyth. 2006. *ACT on Life Not on Anger: The New Acceptance and Commitment Therapy Guide to Problem Anger.* Oakland, CA: New Harbinger Publications.

Forsyth, J. P., and G. H. Eifert. 2018. *Anxiety Happens: 52 Ways to Find Peace of Mind.* Oakland, CA: New Harbinger.

———. 2023. *The Anxiety Happens Guided Journal: Write Your Way to Peace of Mind.* Oakland, CA: New Harbinger Publications.

Goldstein, R. B., S. M. Smith, S. P. Chou, T. D. Saha, J. Jung, H. Zhang, R. P. Pickering, W. J. Ruan, B. Huang, and B. F. Grant. 2016. "The Epidemiology of DSM-5 Posttraumatic Stress Disorder in the United States: Results from the National Epidemiologic Survey on Alcohol and Related Conditions-III." *Social Psychiatry and Psychiatric Epidemiology* 51: 1137–1148.

Goldstein-Piekarski, A., L. Williams, and K. Humphreys. 2016. "A Trans-Diagnostic Review of Anxiety Disorder Comorbidity and the Impact of Multiple Exclusion Criteria on Studying Clinical Outcomes in Anxiety Disorders." *Translational Psychiatry* 6(6): 1–9.

Harris, R. 2008. *The Happiness Trap: How to Stop Struggling and Start Living.* Boston: Trumpeter.

Hayes, S. C. 2004. "Acceptance and Commitment Therapy, Relational Frame Theory, and the Third Wave of Behavioral and Cognitive Therapies." *Behavior Therapy* 35: 639–665.

Hayes, S. C., V. M. Follette, and M. M. Linehan, eds. 2004. *Mindfulness and Acceptance: Expanding the Cognitive-Behavioral Tradition.* New York: Guilford Press.

Hayes, S. C., J. B. Luoma, F. W. Bond, A. Masuda, and J. Lillis. 2006. "Acceptance and Commitment Therapy: Model, Processes, and Outcomes." *Behaviour Research and Therapy* 44(1): 1–25.

Hayes, S. C., K. D. Strosahl, and K. G. Wilson. 2012. *Acceptance and Commitment Therapy: The Process and Practice of Mindful Change,* 2nd ed. New York: Guilford Press.

Hayes, S. C., K. G. Wilson, E. V. Gifford, V. M. Follette, and K. Strosahl. 1996. "Experiential Avoidance and Behavioral Disorders: A Functional Dimensional Approach to Diagnosis and Treatment." *Journal of Consulting and Clinical Psychology* 64: 1152–1168.

Hill, P. L., and N. A. Turiano. 2014. "Purpose in Life as a Predictor of Mortality Across Adulthood." *Psychological Science* 25: 1482–1486.

Hoffmann, D., C. U. Rask, E. Hedman-Lagerlöf, J. S. Jensen, and L. Frostholm. 2021. "Efficacy of Internet-Delivered Acceptance and Commitment Therapy for Severe Health Anxiety: Results from a Randomized, Controlled Trial." *Psychological Medicine* 51(15): 2685–2695.

Ivanova, E., P. Lindner, K. I Ioa Ly, M. Dahlin, K. Vernmark, G. Andersson, and P. Carlbring. 2016. "Guided and Unguided Acceptance and Commitment Therapy for Social Anxiety Disorder and/or Panic Disorder Provided via the Internet and a Smartphone Application: A Randomized Controlled Trial." *Journal of Anxiety Disorders* 44: 27–35.

Kabat-Zinn, J. 1994. *Wherever You Go, There You Are: Mindfulness Meditation in Everyday Life*. New York: Hyperion.

Kessler, R. C., P. Berglund, O. Demler, R. Jin, K. R. Merikangas, and E. E. Walters. 2005. "Lifetime Prevalence and Age-of-Onset Distributions of DSM-IV Disorders in the National Comorbidity Survey Replication." *Archives of General Psychiatry* 62(6): 593–602.

Kessler, R. C., M. Petukhova, N. A. Sampson, A. M. Zaslavsky, and H.-U. Wittchen. 2012. "Twelve-Month and Lifetime Prevalence and Lifetime Morbid Risk of Anxiety and Mood Disorders in the United States." *International Journal of Methods in Psychiatric Research* 21: 169–184.

Konnopka, A., and H. König. 2020. "Economic Burden of Anxiety Disorders: A Systematic Review and Meta-Analysis." *PharmacoEconomics* 38: 25–37.

Leonardo, E. D., and R. Hen. 2006. "Genetics of Affective and Anxiety Disorders." *Annual Review of Psychology* 57: 117–137.

Lesser, E. 2008. *The Seeker's Guide: Making Your Life a Spiritual Adventure*. New York: Ballantine Books.

McKay, M., and C. Sutker. 2007. *Leave Your Mind Behind: The Everyday Practice of Finding Stillness Amid Rushing Thoughts*. Oakland, CA: New Harbinger Publications.

National Center for Health Statistics. US Census Bureau, Household Pulse Survey. 2020–2023. "Anxiety and Depression." https://www.cdc.gov/nchs/covid19/pulse/mental-health.htm.

Newman, M. G., and S. J. Llera. 2011. "A Novel Theory of Experiential Avoidance in Generalized Anxiety Disorder: A Review and Synthesis of Research Supporting a Contrast Avoidance Model of Worry." *Clinical Psychology Review* 31: 371–82.

Nhat Hanh, T. 2001. *Anger: Wisdom for Cooling the Flames*. New York: Riverhead Books, Penguin Putnam.

Orme-Johnson, D. W., and V. A. Barnes. 2014. "Effects of the Transcendental Meditation Technique on Trait Anxiety: A Meta-Analysis of Randomized Controlled Trials." *Journal of Alternative and Complementary Medicine* 20(5): 330–341.

Philip, J., and V. Cherian. 2021. "Acceptance and Commitment Therapy in the Treatment of Obsessive-Compulsive Disorder: A Systematic Review." *Journal of Obsessive-Compulsive and Related Disorders* 28: 1–9.

Ritzert, T., C. R. Berghoff, E. D. Tifft, and J. P. Forsyth, J. P. 2020. "Evaluating ACT Processes in Relation to Outcome in Self-Help Treatment for Anxiety-Related Problems." *Behavior Modification* 44(6): 865–890.

Ritzert, T., J. P. Forsyth, S. C. Sheppard, C. R. Berghoff, J. Boswell, and G. H. Eifert. 2016. "Evaluating the Effectiveness of ACT for Anxiety Disorders in a Self-Help Context: Outcomes from a Randomized Wait-List Controlled Trial." *Behavior Therapy* 47(4): 444–459.

Roth, B. 2022. *Strength in Stillness: The Power of Transcendental Meditation*. New York: Simon and Schuster.

Ruiz, F. J., C. Luciano, C. L. Flórez, J. C. Suárez-Falcón, and V. Cardona-Betancourt. 2020. "A Multiple-Baseline Evaluation of Acceptance and Commitment Therapy Focused on Repetitive Negative Thinking for Comorbid Generalized Anxiety Disorder and Depression." *Frontiers in Psychology* 11: 1–16.

Russo, A. R., J. P. Forsyth, S. C. Sheppard, and R. Promutico. 2009. "Evaluating the Effectiveness of Two Self-Help Workbooks in the Alleviation of Anxious Suffering: What Processes Are Unique to ACT and CBT?" Paper presented at the 43rd annual meeting of the Association for Behavioral and Cognitive Therapies, New York, November.

Salters-Pedneault, K., M. T. Tull, and L. Roemer. 2004. "The Role of Avoidance of Emotional Material in the Anxiety Disorders." *Applied and Preventive Psychology* 11(2): 95–114.

Sedlmeier, P., J. Eberth, M. Schwarz, D. Zimmermann, F. Haarig, S. Jaeger, and S. Kunze. 2012. "The Psychological Effects of Meditation: A Meta-Analysis." *Psychological Bulletin* 138(6): 1139–1171.

Stein, D. J., C. C. W. Lim, A. M. Roest, P. de Jonge, S. Aguilar-Gaxiola, A. Al-Hamzawi, J. Alonso, et al. 2017. "The Cross-National Epidemiology of Social Anxiety Disorder: Data from the World Mental Health Survey Initiative." *BMC Medicine* 15: 1–21.

Strauss, A. Y., Y. Kivity, and J. D. Huppert. 2019. "Emotion Regulation Strategies in Cognitive Behavioral Therapy for Panic Disorder." *Behavior Therapy* 50(3): 659–71.

Swain, J., K. Hancock, C. Hainsworth, and J. Bowman. 2013. "Acceptance and Commitment Therapy in the Treatment of Anxiety: A Systematic Review." *Clinical Psychology Review* 33(8): 965–78.

ter Meulen, W. G., S. Draisma, A. M. van Hemert, R. A. Schoevers, R. W. Kupka, A. T. F. Beekman, and B. W. J. H. Penninx. 2021. "Depressive and Anxiety Disorders in Concert–A Synthesis of Findings on Comorbidity in the NESDA study." *Journal of Affective Disorders* 284: 85–97.

Twohig, M. P., and M. E. Levin. 2017. "Acceptance and Commitment Therapy as a Treatment for Anxiety and Depression: A Review." *Psychiatric Clinics of North America* 40(4): 751–770.

Vahratian, A., S. J. Blumberg, E. P. Terlizzi, and J. S. Schiller. 2021. "Symptoms of Anxiety or Depressive Disorder and Use of Mental Health Care Among Adults During the COVID-19 Pandemic—United States, August 2020–February 2021." *Morbidity and Mortality Weekly Report* 70(13): 490–494.

von Oech, R. 1998. *A Whack on the Side of the Head: How You Can Be More Creative.* New York: Warner Business Books.

Wang, D. A., M. S. Hagger, and N. L. D. Chatzisarantis. 2020. "Ironic Effects of Thought Suppression: A Meta-Analysis." *Perspectives on Psychological Science* 15: 778–793.

Wharton, E., K. S. Edwards, K. Juhasz, and R. D. Walser. 2019. "Acceptance-Based Interventions in the Treatment of PTSD: Group and Individual Pilot Data Using Acceptance and Commitment Therapy." *Journal of Contextual Behavioral Science* 14: 55–64.

Xu, J., S. L. Murphy, K. D. Kochanek, and E. Arias. 2022. "Mortality in the United States, 2021." *National Center for Health Statistics Data Brief* 456: 1–8.

Yadavaia, J. E., S. C. Hayes, and R. Vilardaga. 2014. "Using Acceptance and Commitment Therapy to Increase Self-Compassion: A Randomized Controlled Trial." *Journal of Contextual Behavioral* Science 3(4): 248–257.

Real change *is* possible

For more than fifty years, New Harbinger has published proven-effective self-help books and pioneering workbooks to help readers of all ages and backgrounds improve mental health and well-being, and achieve lasting personal growth. In addition, our spirituality books offer profound guidance for deepening awareness and cultivating healing, self-discovery, and fulfillment.

Founded by psychologist Matthew McKay and Patrick Fanning, New Harbinger is proud to be an independent, employee-owned company. Our books reflect our core values of integrity, innovation, commitment, sustainability, compassion, and trust. Written by leaders in the field and recommended by therapists worldwide, New Harbinger books are practical, accessible, and provide real tools for real change.

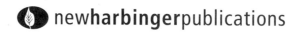 **newharbinger**publications

John P. Forsyth, PhD, is an internationally renowned author and speaker in the fields of acceptance and commitment therapy (ACT), mindfulness practices, and self-development and growth. For over twenty years, his writings, teachings, and research have focused on developing ACT and mindfulness practices to alleviate human suffering, awaken the human spirit, and nurture psychological health and vitality. His personal journey and experience, balanced with practical insights grounded in scientific evidence, offers hope to those wishing to find a path out of suffering and into wholeness. He has coauthored several popular ACT books, including *Acceptance and Commitment Therapy for Anxiety Disorders* for mental health professionals, and several self-help books for the public: *The Mindfulness and Acceptance Workbook for Anxiety*, *Anxiety Happens*, *The Anxiety Happens Guided Journal*, *ACT on Life Not on Anger*, and *Your Life on Purpose*.

Forsyth regularly gives inspirational talks and practical workshops to the public and professionals in the United States and abroad, and offers ACT trainings with his wife at the Kripalu Center for Yoga and Health, the Omega Institute for Holistic Studies, The Esalen Institute, and Cape Cod Institute where he serves as a member of the teaching faculty. He is known to infuse his teaching and trainings with energy, humility, and compassion, and his down-to-earth workshops are consistently praised for their clarity, depth, and utility. Collectively, Forsyth's work has helped foster growing interest in acceptance and mindfulness in psychology, mental health, medicine, and society.

Georg H. Eifert, PhD, is an internationally recognized author, scientist, speaker, and trainer in the use of ACT, an integrative approach balancing mindful acceptance, change, and compassion to foster psychological health and wellness. He is also professor emeritus of psychology at Chapman University in Orange County, CA, where he was previously department chair and associate dean of health sciences. He has won numerous awards for his research, teaching, and writing contributions. He is also a licensed clinical psychologist. As an active developer, researcher, and practitioner of ACT and transcendental meditation, Eifert is coauthor of several popular books, including the highly praised practitioner's treatment guide, *Acceptance and Commitment Therapy for Anxiety Disorders*, as well as several ACT books for the public: *ACT on Life Not on Anger*, *Your Life on Purpose*, and *The Anorexia Workbook*. He has also authored and coauthored several ACT books in German.

Eifert regularly gives workshops and talks around the world, teaching ACT to both the public and professionals to help people end psychological suffering and lead more fulfilling lives. His workshops have been praised as inspiring, humorous, and empowering, and are renowned for their authenticity, clarity, and practical usefulness.

FROM OUR COFOUNDER—

As cofounder of New Harbinger and a clinical psychologist since 1978, I know that emotional problems are best helped with evidence-based therapies. These are the treatments derived from scientific research (randomized controlled trials) that show what works. Whether these treatments are delivered by trained clinicians or found in a self-help book, they are designed to provide you with proven strategies to overcome your problem.

Therapies that aren't evidence-based—whether offered by clinicians or in books—are much less likely to help. In fact, therapies that aren't guided by science may not help you at all. That's why this New Harbinger book is based on scientific evidence that the treatment can relieve emotional pain.

This is important: if this book isn't enough, and you need the help of a skilled therapist, use the following resources to find a clinician trained in the evidence-based protocols appropriate for your problem. And if you need more support—a community that understands what you're going through and can show you ways to cope—resources for that are provided below, as well.

Real help is available for the problems you have been struggling with. The skills you can learn from evidence-based therapies will change your life.

Matthew McKay, PhD
Cofounder, New Harbinger Publications

If you need a therapist, the following organization can help you find a therapist trained in acceptance and commitment therapy (ACT).

Association for Contextual Behavioral Science (ACBS)
please visit www.contextualscience.org and click on Find an ACT Therapist.

For additional support for patients, family, and friends, contact the following:

Anxiety and Depression Association of American (ADAA)
please visit www.adaa.org

National Alliance on Mental Illness (NAMI)
please visit www.nami.org

Also by the Authors

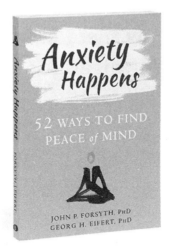

This powerful, portable guide is packed with
52 in-the-moment mindfulness strategies you can use
anytime, anywhere to cultivate calm and peace of mind.

978-1684031108 / US $14.95

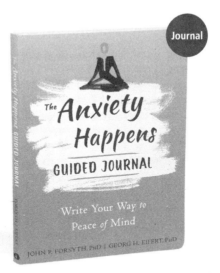

Pick up your pen and put anxiety in its place with
this soothing guided journal—full of simple ways
to unwind and calm your worries.

978-1648482113 / US $18.95

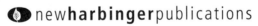 **newharbinger**publications

1-800-748-6273 / newharbinger.com

Did you know there are **free tools** you can download for this book?

Free tools are things like **worksheets**, **guided meditation exercises**, and **more** that will help you get the most out of your book.

You can download free tools for this book— whether you bought or borrowed it, in any format, from any source—from the New Harbinger website. All you need is a NewHarbinger.com account. Just use the URL provided in this book to view the free tools that are available for it. Then, click on the "download" button for the free tool you want, and follow the prompts that appear to log in to your NewHarbinger.com account and download the material.

You can also save the free tools for this book to your **Free Tools Library** so you can access them again anytime, just by logging in to your account! Just look for this button on the book's free tools page.

+ Save this to my free tools library